Adolescents and Sex

The handbook for professionals working with young people

Sarah Bekaert
Development Nurse
City and Hackney Young People's Services

Forewords by

Ann McPherson

and

Ceri Evans

Radcliffe Publishing

Radcliffe Publishing Ltd
18 Marcham Road
Abingdon
Oxon OX14 1AA
United Kingdom

www.radcliffe-oxford.com
Electronic catalogue and worldwide online ordering facility.

British Library Cataloguing in Publication Data

A catalogue record for this book is available from the British Library.

ISBN 1 85775 880 3

Typeset by Aarontype Ltd, Easton, Bristol
Printed and bound by TJ International Ltd, Padstow, Cornwall

Contents

Foreword

The expression of sexuality in the teenage years depends on many different things. There is the inevitability of the physiology and that the hormones will come into play at puberty. There is the balance between the sexual and the reproductive drive. Whereas sexuality is being made available, and in some cases promoted, to a younger and younger age group, at the same time sexuality leading to reproduction is being demoted. There is the influence of the media and advertising who know that, like violence, sex sells, and sell it hard. And there are also the other cultural influences including peer pressure and religion. It is therefore not surprising that some young people find themselves confused by the different messages.

But where does the health professional enter the sexual area? Information and provision of services are two key areas where we (they) have a role. But even here there are confusions as research shows that young people want different aspects of information about sex from different people. They want relationship information primarily from their parents, the basic biology from schools and information on contraception and sexually transmitted infections from health professionals.

In order to give really good advice over a relatively small area of knowledge that young people require in this field, health professionals need a wide range of knowledge about not only contraception and sexually transmitted infections but also these other areas to give balance and to put the information in the appropriate context.

This book by Sarah Bekaert covers all aspects that any health professional working in this area needs. It provides the broad sweep and the detail as well as reflecting the complexity and breadth of the subject. There is information about the changes at puberty, how to engage young people, the legal issues, contraception and sexually transmitted infections, as well as ideas on how to deliver the service to 'get it right' for the young people who use it. There are no quick fixes and many different models. None of us want young people to have sex or get pregnant in their early teens or before they are emotionally ready. We all know ambition is one of the best forms of contraception. Unfortunately health professionals alone can do little to bring this about but we can make sure that what we do and should provide to help this end, we do well and in a teenage friendly way.

Ann McPherson
General Practitioner
Co-author of the best selling *Teenage Health Freak* series
Chair of the RCGP Adolescent Task Force
November 2004

Foreword

This is a well-timed book – almost every day the press carries reports of rising numbers of unplanned pregnancies and sexually transmitted infections in young people. This is almost certainly down to the ill-effects of young adults having little or no access to good information about sexual health and relationships.

For our young people to have competence in their sexual lives and confidence in the services we are offering them, as professionals, we need to listen to what they are saying and offer services tailored to their needs. We are accountable to and for our young people and our provision for their sexual good health should be one of our priorities.

Young people should be actively encouraged and welcomed into sexual health clinics, GP surgeries and family planning services. School nurses should be well informed and promote good sexual health, and SRE and PHSE should be a statutory right in schools. Until sexual health becomes a priority in all these situations we will continue to experience unacceptable rates of sexually transmitted infections.

This book gives us all the chance to start as we mean to go on – by giving us practical and useful information and tools to inform, change and protect a generation who need our unwavering and judgement-free support.

I hope every statutory and voluntary organisation that has contact with young people gets a copy of this book – and uses it.

Ceri Evans
Senior Health Adviser
West London Centre for Sexual Health
Chelsea and Westminster Healthcare NHS Trust
November 2004

Preface

Working with young people is exciting and rewarding, yet can present many challenges. Sexual health and contraceptive issues with this group often raise legal, ethical and sometimes child protection concerns.

I am a paediatric nurse working in a multidisciplinary team in Hackney, East London. We run young people's sexual health and contraception clinics and carry out health promotion outreach work in schools and youth groups.

As a team we have a wealth of knowledge in areas such as communication, working with marginalised groups and outreach work. This book aims to communicate this knowledge in an appealing and useful manner to professionals who come into contact with young people.

Setting up young people's clinics has involved a great deal of resourcing and networking for up-to-date and relevant information to underpin practice. This text brings together, in a quick reference format, the information on legal and ethical issues, teenage pregnancy, sexual health, contraception and sexually transmitted infections. I have included a step-by-step guide to setting up a young person's clinic and information on outreach work with young people.

The text aims to be informative and practical. For those who have more time or if a particular area is of interest, there are signposts for further reading and suggested resources.

Sarah Bekaert
November 2004

About the author

Sarah Bekaert is a development nurse for City and Hackney Young People's Services, where she combines a specialist interest in adolescent care and sexual health.

She gained her first degree in French Studies at Manchester University and subsequently worked for the relief and development agency Tearfund. She then trained as a paediatric nurse at St Bartholomew's School of Nursing and Midwifery and has worked in paediatrics, school nursing and practice nursing – all in the borough of Hackney. Since qualifying she obtained a BSc in Nursing and is currently undertaking a MSc in Community Gynaecology and Reproductive Health Care at Warwick University. She is an associate member of the Faculty of Family Planning and Reproductive Health Care and an assessor for the Royal College of Nursing distance-learning course in sexual health skills.

Aged 32, she is married to photographer Geoff Crawford and has an eight-month-old daughter.

Acknowledgements

The idea for this handbook arose from a collaborative project to set up a young person's sexual health clinic between City and Hackney Young People's Services and Homerton Hospital Genito-urinary Medicine Services. I would like to thank my work colleagues, Alison White, Maurice Cunningham and Gwyneth Hearn, for their enthusiasm and expertise.

I would also like to thank Christine Twomey, Suzanne Everett and especially my mum, Enid Frost, for being inspirational role models; Gillian Nineham at Radcliffe for her support and encouragement; and my husband, Geoff, for his proofreading skills and unfailing patience.

For Ruby-May

Introduction

This book has been written with the intention of providing a quick reference guide for professionals who provide sexual health and contraceptive services for young people. It is designed to be read as a whole, but recognising a health professional's workload, each chapter stands alone and can be dipped into to address a specific query.

Each chapter tackles a particular area relating to young people's sexual health and contraception. Starting with useful background knowledge, it moves on to practical information regarding periods, contraceptive methods, pregnancy, abortion and sexually transmitted infections and dispels some of the associated common myths.

The book includes practical advice and information on reaching marginalised groups such as young people with learning difficulties and disability and young people in care. A chapter is devoted to legal issues and ethical concerns, such as consent and child protection, which arise when dealing with young people and sexual relations. Finally there is a description of how to set up a young people's clinic – the policies required and procedures and practical suggestions for outreach work.

The book's primary aim is to provide practical information to inform practice with young people in the area of sexual health and contraception; however, each chapter includes a reference list for those who wish to further explore a particular area.

Each chapter uses scenarios and illustrations to stimulate critical thought and may be used as teaching materials. In addition, a list of useful resources is provided for each subject area.

Health professionals often see young people as a difficult and challenging group. This book will help those professionals to meet the challenge of working with young people in the area of sexual health and contraception with confidence and understanding.

CHAPTER 1

The teenage years

OK, so I've got my GCSEs this year, but I am 15 and mum won't let me go to Sharon's party this weekend! I just have to go because Mark will be there and I've fancied him for ages ... It's not fair, everyone else is going. Anyhow, I haven't got anything to wear anyway, and I'm breaking out. My period must be coming ...

What is adolescence?

The teenage years are a fun but anxious time as the young person becomes more independent and explores their identity. At the same time their body is going through great change that can be both exciting and scary.

The teenage years are often referred to as adolescence. But what exactly is adolescence? It is difficult to find agreement on when this stage of life begins and ends, and it depends on who is trying to define it.

Age

The World Health Organization defines adolescence as being between the ages of 10 and 20. This is an abrupt and inadequate starting and ending point as it doesn't account for variations in individual development; girls often start developing earlier than boys, with boys catching up towards the end of the teenage years. Some start developing earlier than age 10 and some finish later than 20.

Legal definitions

There are no clear legal definitions for adolescence either. Exactly when a young person can legally assume an adult role is confusing. People under 18 are considered to be minors yet can marry aged 16 and drive at 17. It is recognised in common law that a young person under 16 may be capable of making their own decisions regarding their health. This followed the Gillick case in 1986 that debated the ability of under-16s to seek confidential contraceptive advice from their doctor.[1] From this case came the Fraser Guidelines (after Lord Fraser, who presided over the case) that are now used as criteria for assessing a young person's ability to make decisions regarding their healthcare, particularly in contraception and sexual health matters. This is discussed in more detail in Chapter 3.

Thought processes

The psychologist Piaget claimed that maturation in reasoning ability coincides with adolescence (*see* Box 1.1).[2] However, he also said that this may be achieved later in life and that some people do not achieve this stage (formal operations). So this ability may emerge during adolescence but it is not exclusive to it. Thus we cannot define adolescence by thought-processing ability alone.

Biology

Adolescence is a time of rapid physiological change and growth. Puberty can occur at any time between the ages of nine and 16. It is not possible to identify a definite start and end to this growth spurt – it is different for every individual. Furthermore, there is a marked difference in the age at which puberty begins in girls and boys. Periods usually start sometime between the ages of 10 and 16 in girls and testicular growth is usually complete between ages 13 and 17 in boys. Table 1.1 summarises the physical maturation of boys and girls.[3]

Psychology

The psychologist Erikson describes adolescence as a period of identity formation.[4] Young people begin to seek independence from parents, start to identify with peer groups, explore their own belief systems and generally begin to form their own identity. Yet this is a continuous process throughout life and although defining identity is distinctive during adolescence, it is not exclusive to it.

Box 1.1   Piaget's stages of cognitive development[2]

Sensori-motor (birth–2 years)
• Differentiates self from objects
• Begins to act intentionally
• Realises that things continue to exist even when not in view (object permanence)

Pre-operational (2–7 years)
• Develops language, recognises images and words
• Has difficulty taking the viewpoint of others (egocentric thought)
• Sorts objects by single feature only, e.g. all red blocks regardless of shape

Concrete operational (7–11 years)
• Thinks logically about objects and events
• Understands idea of weight and numbers
• Sorts objects according to several features

Formal operations (11 years and up)
• Can think logically about abstract propositions and test hypotheses systematically

Table 1.1   The physical maturation of boys and girls[3]

Girls	Physical changes
Average age 11 years	Breast development: stage 1 – no glandular development stage 2 – breast bud change stage 3 – breast bud stage with nipple protrusion stage 4 – nipple and areola form a mound distinct from breast tissue
Average age 14–16 years	stage 5 – mature breast
One year after breast bud development	Pubic hair growth: stage 1 – no pubic hair stage 2 – sparse hair growth along labia stage 3 – coarse hair growth spreading sparsely over symphysis pubis stage 4 – growth increases but does not extend to medial surface of thighs stage 5 – adult pattern of growth, extending to medial aspects of thighs Axillary hair growth
One year after stage 2 pubic hair development 10–15 years	Menarche – initial cycles may be anovulatory, ovulation begins within two years Height increases – growth spurt at around 12 years Increased apocrine gland secretion may result in acne

Boys	Physical changes
10–13 years – average 11 years	Genital development: stage 1 – no enlargement of testes and penis stage 2 – enlargement of testes, scrotum becomes more pigmented, no enlargement of penis stage 3 – penis enlarges in length, continued enlargement of testes stage 4 – penis grows in length and width, glans development, enlargement of testes
Average age 15–16 years	stage 5 – mature genital
10–13 years with stage 2 development	Pubic hair growth
14–15 years	Facial hair growth, voice changes, height increases, growth spurt at approximately 14 years
Approximately three years after stage 2 development	Ejaculation possible, mature sperm between approximately 14 and 16 years

A Western invention

There doesn't appear to be a clear definition of what adolescence is and when it occurs. Some sociologists would go so far as to claim adolescence is artificially created; it has occurred because of the increasing demands of a complex modern society where young people require knowledge of more things to be able to cope with adult life, and as a result there needs to be a time to process and assimilate all this information. This would appear true as many developing countries do not have a transitional period between child and adulthood. It would also account for the fact that there are characteristics that are common yet not exclusive to adolescence.

The tasks of adolescence

It is difficult to pin down what adolescence is. It is all of the above yet none exclusively. However, there are issues that young people typically grapple with during the teenage years. Sociologists have tried to identify the common issues that present during this time. For example, Havinghurst[5] describes 'tasks of adolescence' (*see* Box 1.2) that should be achieved if an adolescent is to function effectively in adult society.

Forming a clear identity

The need to find an identity is a common driving force for young people; they often identify with certain reference groups. These may be typified by outward appearance such as clothes or hairstyles, or activities they engage in like church groups, music genres, etc. Peer relationships are formed within these groups.

Independence from parents is explored when forming an individual identity. Often 'parental' or 'adult' guidance is rejected as the young person wants to explore issues themselves, with disbelief that anyone could have gone through what they are experiencing! The choices a young person has to make – which group to belong to, belief systems, career, emerging sexuality – can be overwhelming. Often they move from one idea to another as they explore the possibilities. This can be confusing for the adults who observe these inconsistencies.

Box 1.2   Havinghurst's 'tasks of adolescence'[5]

- Forming a clear identity.
- Developing a personal value system.
- Gaining independence from parents.
- Achieving financial and social independence.
- Accepting a new body image.
- Developing relationships with members of both sexes.
- Developing cognitive skills and the ability to think abstractly.
- Developing the ability to control one's behaviour according to socially acceptable norms and taking responsibility for one's own behaviour.

However, it is important to support the young person as they explore their identity. Consistency from adults in their lives provides trustworthy role models.

Individual rates of physical development can influence whether a young person is included in groups. A young person who is developing at a slower rate than his or her peers may still appear childlike and find it difficult to be included in the more 'advanced' groups. It can also be difficult to explore your identity if you are unable to become independent from parents and carers due to a disability – this will be discussed more fully in Chapter 8.

Box 1.3   Bullying

Non-acceptance by the peer group can result in bullying which causes psychological distress for the young person. Professionals working with young people should be aware that this may be an underlying problem in a young person's life.

What is bullying? Bullying includes a wide variety of behaviours, but all involve a person or a group repeatedly trying to harm someone who is weaker or more vulnerable. It can involve direct attacks such as hitting, threatening or intimidating, maliciously teasing and taunting, name calling, making sexual remarks, and stealing or damaging a person's belongings; or it can involve more subtle, indirect attacks such as the spreading of rumours or encouraging others to reject or exclude someone.

Bullying can lead young people to feel tense, anxious, and afraid. If bullying continues for some time, it can affect self-esteem and self-worth. It can increase social isolation, leading victims to become withdrawn and depressed, anxious and insecure. Years later, long after the bullying has stopped, adults who were bullied as young people have higher levels of depression and poorer self-esteem than other adults.

Developing a personal value system

The young person starts to develop thoughts and actions about what is right and wrong rather than simply accepting parental beliefs. As they expand their social circles every young person will be faced with changing and sometimes conflicting values and standards of behaviour. Typically they will look to their peer groups to gain insight into how to behave. This can be complicated by conflicting approaches of peer groups and the young person's inexperience in making moral decisions. This may result in what the adult world would call delinquent behaviour or rebellious behaviour yet is often simply experimentation with new possibilities. Adults should present sound consistent values to young people. The young people will observe this and these values will be incorporated into their decision-making processes. Value systems adopted can be simplistic, but equally valid in a complex society.

Gaining independence from parents

Parents will usually promote independence as a young person grows older. This depends on the parent–child relationship before adolescence. If the relationship has been overprotective the young person will have difficulty exploring their own identity. Equally, some young people may find it difficult to cope with the demands of being independent and will reject the opportunity, keeping 'childlike' behaviours.

A young person may move between adult and childlike behaviour, which can be confusing for parents/carers and health professionals. For example, an expanding social life can be dependent on parental transport and funding or a developing sexual relationship may not go hand in hand with a responsible approach to contraception and safe sex.

Achieving financial and social independence

The social environment provides a filter through which the adolescent perceives the world. As they grow older they select and interpret these perceptions. A nurturing familial and social environment will support this. As a young person gets older parents may engender a practical approach to saving and budgeting by providing an allowance. Young people can take on part-time work and begin to have financial independence. This can be the cause of great conflict between parents/carers and young people; they have been used to parents providing clothes and recreational activities, yet as they grow older their tastes become more expensive and they perceive needs where parents may not! Conflict may also arise where young people prioritise casual work over study, preferring to be cash rich currently rather than investing in preparation for future security.

Some groups, such as young people with illness or disability, may experience problems in achieving social and financial independence from parents. They may be restricted in their ability to travel independently or by the jobs that are available to them.

Accepting a new body image

Adolescents have little control over their changing bodies. With puberty come spots, sweat and body hair. To successfully accept a new body image they need to be able to adapt to these changes. Some young people can develop preoccupations with body image that may result in problems such as anorexia nervosa and bulimia. It is not clear why some young people develop these problems and others do not, however it could be due to culturally defined messages that are portrayed by the media about the 'ideal' body shape and weight. Young people may feel undue pressure to conform to these unnatural 'norms'. Some young people may not be ready for imminent adulthood and develop eating behaviours to try to stay thin and childlike.

Adolescents who have been sexually abused may be particularly confused about their emerging sexuality and sexual identity. An adult appearance may be associated with negative feelings. The young person may need support to re-evaluate these feelings and learn to develop healthy and fulfilling sexual relationships.

Meanwhile, a hormonal roller-coaster can cause mood swings, volatile behaviour and a general lack of control over emotions. This can be an unpredictable and difficult time for young people.

Developing relationships with members of both sexes

Peer relationships become increasingly important during adolescence. Their role is often to provide a support mechanism and a reference group with which the young person can begin to identify. At first it is typical for a young person to form same-sex friendships, then in the later teens pairing off is common. Young people may struggle with issues such as sexuality, whether they are attractive, and how to act in relationships.

Developing cognitive skills and abstract thought

At the same time as all these physical changes are occurring for a young person, complexity of thought processes is developing. An ability to give consideration to a range of consequences and to reason develops, leading to logical and systematic decision making. However, this is an on-going process and the teenage years are characterised by egocentric thought: the notion that what they are thinking and experiencing is completely new and unique to them. It is important to bear in mind when working with a group of young people that they will all be at different stages in this process.

Developing behaviour control according to socially acceptable norms and taking responsibility for behaviour

Usually the peer group provides the main reference for behavioural choices for a young person. Sometimes the peer group influence may override parents, and may be seen as rebellious behaviour. Self-esteem and self-confidence influence a young person's ability to make independent behavioural choices. However, the strong desire for belonging can influence a young person's choice of behaviour within a peer group. Sometimes the peer group can exert great influence on the young person. It is very important for the young person to feel accepted and hence to conform to the group norm. This can range from choice of clothing to more risky behaviours such as drug taking.

Peer pressure: Stanley Milgram's obedience experiments

The following is an illustration of the extremes to which peer pressure can lead people. In the 1950s, the psychologist Stanley Milgram[6] wanted to see how an individual conscience responds to authority. He devised a series of experiments to see how far individuals would go in inflicting pain on another human being when told to do so by an 'authority figure'.

Forty males aged 20–50 years were studied. They were asked to give someone they couldn't see and had never met increasingly powerful electric shocks whenever they answered a memory question wrongly. The person that they were 'shocking' was actually an actor – but they didn't know this. Whenever a subject didn't want to give a 'shock' the scientist alongside them repeated that the

Table 1.2 Milestones of adolescence

Milestone	Consequences for the young person	Effect on the family
Milestones of early adolescence, 11–14 years		
Worries about appearance of developing body	Self-consciousness	Parents, teachers, peers may see this as selfishness
Hormonal changes	General moodiness. Boys who were previously gentle and easy-going may become more aggressive. Acne may appear in both boys and girls	Surliness may be hard to live with and accommodate
Asserts independence and may feel an individual, not just a family member	Experiments with dress, speech, manners, etc. in an attempt to find a separate identity	Parents may feel rejected and have difficulty in accepting the child's independence
Rebellious defiant behaviour	Rudeness, demands more freedom	Interaction with the child needs to be carefully managed if relationships are to be maintained
Friends become important	Wants to identify with friends by clothes, hairstyle, music, etc.	Parents may be irritated by apparent conformity and financial demands
Milestones of middle adolescence, 15–16 years		
Becomes less self-absorbed, develops greater flexibility to compromise	More composed, tolerant, accepts that other opinions can be valid	Easier to live with, more cooperative
Experiments continually to find comfortable self-image	Likely to experiment with drugs, alcohol or cigarettes	Anxious about risks, parents must decide how and when to set limits
Develops values, personal morality	Questions and maybe rejects ideas and values absorbed from school and family	Conflict if important family values are rejected
Accepts own sexuality, forms sexual relations involving new feelings	Starts dating, guards privacy and may seem secretive, forms short relationships	Parental anxiety about safety may be seen as intrusive

Milestone	Consequences for the young person	Effect on the family
Lasting relationships	Wants to spend less time with family and more with friends	Parents resent their home being treated as a hotel
Intellectual development, wider awareness and interests, able to think in abstract terms and deal with hypothetical questions	Questions things previously taken for granted, likes to discuss and debate issues	Parents learn to know their offspring
Becomes physically and socially adventurous, wants to travel	Takes risks and may suffer accidents	Fear that intervening may antagonise offspring

Milestones of late adolescence, 17–18 years

Idealistic	Attempts to find social or political cause; religious cults and beliefs very attractive	Distress at apparent rejection of own culture
Involvement with life/work and outside relationships	Must learn to cope with stresses which inevitably follow; may want to be socially with friends rather than family	Parents' wish to protect child may cause friction; parents may appreciate their new found freedom
Seeks financial and emotional independence	Anxiety about the future may affect confidence and moods	Parents may supply financial support even though child is not emotionally dependent; may result in friction and unease
More able to form stable sexual relationships	Likely to have steady boy/girlfriend	Worry about early commitment
Feels on equal terms with adults in the family	Feelings of superior insight	Parents may feel condescended to and resent this
Almost ready to become independent adult	May leave home/university to find own living arrangements	Parental relationships may require adjustment

experiment 'demanded' that they continue and told them they were not responsible for the consequences. The subject could not see the 'student', but could hear the responses, which were frequently incorrect, as well as the screams that accompanied the simulated electric shocks. Two-thirds of the volunteers were fully obedient, continually administering the maximum 450 volt shocks, even after the students' screams were replaced by an ominous silence.

The frightening results were that most people did what they were told to do, regardless of the consequences. When you hear the account of Milgram's experiments you agree that disobedience is the correct course. People who have not taken part in the study assume that of course they would refuse. Yet Milgram's experiment shows that internal values seem to have little correlation with actual behaviour.

Table 1.2 summarises the tasks of adolescence and describes the age at which certain issues come to the fore.[7]

The young person typically explores many areas of increasing independence: decision making, choosing friends, forming an identity and developing sexuality. Ideally, young people are able to experiment and make mistakes within a supportive family network and social environment. This is not always possible as these relationships may restrict or allow too much independence, resulting in rebellious or even delinquent behaviour.

Risk-taking behaviour

As a young person explores the adult world they may engage in risk-taking behaviour. Box 1.4 shows statistics that illustrate typical detrimental health behaviours.

Box 1.4   Adolescent health concerns

Smoking
Thirteen per cent of 11–15 year-olds reported that they smoked.[8]

Alcohol
More than 40% of boys and girls aged 16 report weekly alcohol consumption of an average of 3.4 units per boy and 1.6 units per girl. Binge drinking, an excessive intake of alcohol at one time, is an increasing problem.[8]

Drugs and solvents
Nine per cent of 12–13 year-olds said they had taken illegal drugs or solvents, rising to 30% of 14–15 year-olds and 37% of 15–16 year-olds.[8]

Pregnancy
In 2000, 62.2 in every 1000 15–16 year-olds became pregnant in England and Wales.[9]

Sexually transmitted infections
In 1995–97, 16–19 year-olds had the highest rate of increase in gonorrhoea, with a 45% increase in new cases. Diagnoses for chlamydia rose by 53%.[10]

Depression

Suicide amongst teenagers and young adults has increased threefold since 1970.

   Ninety per cent of suicide amongst teenagers had a diagnosable mental illness, depression being the most common.

   In 1996, suicide was the fourth biggest killer of 10–14-year-olds, and the third biggest killer of 15–24 year-olds.[11]

Self-harm

Ten per cent of teenagers aged 15 and 16 have deliberately self-harmed. The majority (greater than 64%) of those who self-harm cut themselves. Girls are nearly four times more likely to self-harm than boys. The most common reason given was to find relief from a terrible situation.[12]

Weight

In Britain, it is thought that up to 5% of girls are anorexic.[13]

Substance abuse

Young people tend to live in the here and now and can find it difficult to attach significance to how their current behaviour will influence their health in future years. They have a sense of infallibility, the 'it'll never happen to me' approach. Hence young people often experiment with behaviours that may be detrimental to their health in the future, such as smoking, binge drinking and drug taking.

   Smoking has future negative consequences such as increased asthma, bronchitis and even cancer. Smoking when pregnant can lead to the baby having a low birth weight and increased susceptibility to illness. Alcohol can impair reaction times and increase the likelihood of accidents as well as reduce the ability to make reasoned decisions that leads to other risky behaviour such as unprotected sexual intercourse. Long-term use of alcohol can lead to liver cirrhosis. Similarly, other drugs can increase accidents and risk-taking behaviours as well as the Russian roulette chance of having an adverse reaction to a substance in an illegal drug.

   The following example that made headline news is an example of teenage risk-taking behaviour under the influence of drugs and peer pressure:

Monday 14 July 2003

Detention for teen-death driver

A 17-year-old boy has been sent to a detention centre for two years for causing the death of his best friend in a car crash in Cumbria. He has also been banned from driving for four years.

   The teenager was 16 and under the influence of cannabis when the car he was driving crashed into a tanker between Carlisle and Kirkbamton. Four of his friends were passengers and one of them, 14-year-old Rodney Hanlon, was killed. Two others, including the driver, were seriously injured. He admitted causing Rodney Hanlon's death by careless driving while unfit through drugs.

> Carlisle Crown Court heard the teenager had never driven a car before but was persuaded to get behind the wheel by his friends. The youths had been smoking cannabis in a church car park.
>
> The judge was given details of what he called the boy's 'exceedingly difficult and deprived childhood'. But he said he had no option but to impose a two-year detention and training order.[14]

Sexual health

In recent years young people have become sexually active at a younger age:

- the age at which the majority of 16–19 year-olds today first have heterosexual sexual intercourse is 16
- almost 30% of young men and almost 26% of young women report having had intercourse before their 16th birthday. By the age of 20 the vast majority of young people today will have had sex.[9]

Sexual intercourse at a younger age and poor condom use have led to increased rates of sexually transmitted infections (STIs) in the teenage group. The Government has responded to the general increase in STIs with the National Strategy for Sexual Health and HIV.[15] In summary, it recommends the promotion of sexual health and of mainstream sexual health services to dissipate the stigma that is commonly associated with STIs. This will be covered in greater detail in Chapter 6.

Contraception and pregnancy

Contraception and sexual health are particular focus areas for professionals working with young people. The United Kingdom (UK) has the highest teenage pregnancy rates in Western Europe. The Government has recognised the problem and set up a specific working group, called the Teenage Pregnancy Unit, to formulate strategies to tackle teen pregnancy. The resultant Teenage Pregnancy Strategy[10] outlines targets for the reduction in teen pregnancy rates of 40–60% by 2010. Teenage pregnancy can result in what the Government calls 'social exclusion'; reduced opportunity to socialise, carry on with education, find work and a resulting poverty cycle for young parents. There is also an increased incidence of childhood illness and accidents in children born to teenage parents. Issues surrounding teenage pregnancy will be covered in greater detail in Chapter 4.

Sources of health information for young people

The challenge for professionals working with young people is to engage them in positive health behaviours so that beneficial health foundations can be laid for future years. It is essential that young people receive health information, and in this case sexual health information, from a reliable source to equip them with the correct knowledge to make informed decisions. However, health professionals are rarely the first port of call for this information. In one survey of young people, GPs

Table 1.3 From where do young people get their sexual health information?[16]

Magazines	70%
Friends	63%
TV	54%
GPs	14%
Parents	14%

ranked alongside parents as people they would go to for sexual health advice, with magazines, friends and the television being preferred resources (*see* Table 1.3).[16]

What puts teens off seeking professional advice?

More often than not young people seek contraceptive and sexual health advice after they have become sexually active. It would be ideal if they did so when starting a new relationship, before they become sexually active.

There are several common reasons young people give when asked what puts them off seeking advice sooner. When interviewed in a local surgery about what would put them off coming, the following themes emerged:

• *Waiting.* They do not like having to wait, for example when appointments are running late, or having to book appointments several weeks in advance.

'Waiting too much to see a doctor' (male aged 17)
'Waiting time, too many people' (female aged 17)
'Sitting in a waiting room feeling like people are looking at you' (female aged 14)
'Can't get an appointment that easily (have to wait)' (female aged 17)
'Sometimes you have to wait longer than you are supposed to for a doctor' (female aged 15)
'You sometimes have to wait over a week if you want an appointment with your choice of doctor' (male aged 17)

• *Confidentiality.* They are concerned about confidentiality and worry that if they share something personal, doctors and nurses will then tell their parents. Young people also worry that receptionists will unwittingly reveal information about their attendance to family members or that health professionals will contact their parents. Reassurance about confidentiality should be both written and verbal, and should specifically mention under-16s.

> 'Might tell parents I've been in' (female aged 14)
> 'Family members finding out about personal problems' as well as 'So many people from my estate go to the same surgery' was off-putting for one male aged 15

- *Lack of confidence*. They are not sure what to expect and are not confident in a new environment.

> 'Feeling stupid, embarrassment' (female aged 14)
> 'I don't really know my doctor on a personal level so this makes me a little shy, so I take my mum!' (female aged 17)

They also worry about how staff will react to them, and whether they will disapprove of their sexual activity.

> 'Patronising doctors and nurses' (female aged 14)
> 'Slightly intimidating' (male aged 17)

- *The environment*. The waiting room environment is important to this age group. It reveals what the service thinks of young people and whether it actively welcomes them.

> 'Good magazines [required]' (male aged 17)
> 'Unclean toilets and tramps' were off-putting for one female 17-year-old
> 'Too crowdy most of the time' (female aged 15)
> 'Sick people' (male aged 16)
> The 'likelihood of catching an illness in the waiting room' (male aged 17)
> In response to the prompt to 'write down something that puts you off coming to the surgery', one young female aged 14 simply wrote 'the ATMOSPHERE'

The young people's responses showed common concerns regarding confidentiality, feeling judged by staff members and a lack of confidence in seeking health advice. They also raised issues such as enabling a young person to be seen quickly and considering whether the environment is welcoming to this age group. In addition, young people may make it to a consultation but not feel confident to reveal the real issue, and come away with their problem undiscussed and unresolved. These are all important considerations when setting up a young person's service or simply looking at whether a facility is young people friendly.[17] This is discussed in more detail in Chapter 9.

Summary

It is difficult to define what and when adolescence is, although there appear to be characteristics that are common to adolescence such as changing appearance, growing identity and independence as well as experimentation with adult behaviour and risk taking. The degree of maturity can vary from individual to individual and issues such as peer pressure and bullying should be borne in mind when dealing with a young person's sexual health and contraceptive needs.

References

1   Gillick *v* West Norfolk and Wisbech Area Health Authority (1985) 1 AC 12, 184 G.

2   Piaget J (1954) *The Construction of Reality in the Child*. Basic books, New York. In: Taylor J and Muller D (1995) *Nursing Adolescents: research and psychological perspectives*. Blackwell Science, Oxford.

3   Fuller J and Schaller-Ayers J (1994) *Health Assessment: a nursing approach*. JB Lippencott, Baltimore, MD. In: Blackie C, Gregg R and French D (1998) Promoting health in young people. *Nursing Standard.* **12** (36): 39–46.

4   Erikson E (1965) *Childhood and Society*. Penguin, Harmondsworth. In: Taylor J and Muller D (1995) *Nursing Adolescents: research and psychological perspectives*. Blackwell Science, Oxford.

5   Havinghurst RJ (1952) *Developmental Tasks and Education*. David McKay, New York.

6   Milgram S (1963) Behavioural study of obedience. *Journal of Abnormal and Social Psychology.* **67**: 371–8. Also in: Gross R (1992) *Psychology: the science of mind and behaviour* (2e). Hodder and Stoughton, London.

7   Fenwick E and Smith T (1993) Adolescence: the survival guide for parents. Dorling Kindersley, London. In: Blackie C, Gregg R and French D (1998) Promoting health in young people. *Nursing Standard.* **12** (36): 39–46.

8   Walker Z, Townsend JL, Bell J and Marshall S (1999) An opportunity for teenage health promotion in general practice: an assessment of current provision and needs. *Health Education Journal.* **58**: 218–27.

9   Brook Advisory (2003) *Teenage Conceptions: statistics and trends*. www.brook. org.uk/content/fact2_TeenageConceptions.pdf

10   Social Exclusion Unit (1999) *Teenage Pregnancy Strategy*. HMSO, London.

11   *Teen Depression* (2004). www.clinicaldepression.co.uk/Depression_informa tion/teen.htm

12   Samaritans (2003) *Youth and Self-harm Perspectives*. Samaritans, London.

13   www.bbc.co.uk/birmingham/teens/2002/08/anorexia/shtml

14   http://news.bbc.co.uk/1/hi/england/cumbria/3060143.stm (14/07/03)

15   Department of Health (2001) *National Strategy for Sexual Health and HIV*. HMSO, London.

16   Lemp H, Rink E and Harris T (1998) Sexual health information in primary health care. *British Journal of Community Nursing.* **3** (10): 483–8.

17   Bekaert S (2003) Developing adolescent services in general practice. *Nursing Standard.* **17** (36): 33–6.

Resources

- Taylor J and Muller D (1995) *Nursing Adolescents: research and psychological perspectives*. Blackwell Science, Oxford. This concise textbook gives a good overview of adolescence. Although written from a nursing perspective, the information is useful for many disciplines.

- www.teenagepregnancyunit.gov.uk
  Government website with Teenage Pregnancy Strategy and associated documents, press releases and resources.

- www.doh.gov.uk/nshs/strategy.htm
  Full text version of the Government's National Strategy for Sexual Health and HIV.

- www.bullying.co.uk
  Help and advice for victims of bullying, their parents and school.

CHAPTER 2

Engaging young people

Adolescents are a specific client group, requiring specialist skills to cater for their needs. It is helpful to have knowledge of young people's development, both cognitive and physiological, for effective communication, and an idea of the issues influencing their thought processes and actions. However, professionals working with young people can draw on general communication skills for effective interaction: listening skills, observation, the use of body language, the ability to assess understanding and choosing the best medium in which to communicate.

This chapter looks at how communication with young people can be enhanced. Professionals working with young people should ask themselves: are we engaging all groups in the community? Are there groups in the community that need specialist provision? Is the service we provide at the best time and in the best place for young people to access? Are the premises welcoming to young people? Consultation skills should be examined. Does the young person feel valued and listened to? Have they understood the information given? Do the media we use attract young people to our service? It then covers needs assessment, the consultation process, the clinic environment, consultation skills, advertising a service and outreach work with young people.

Groundwork
Needs assessment

A needs assessment is the first step in setting up a service for young people. Community networking is helpful to find out what is being done locally for young people and what plans are proposed. Is your service already being provided in the local community? Could you work in partnership with other groups? Are other people hoping to set up a similar service and, if so, would joint working be possible? Where is the best location for the service? A health centre can medicalise services – perhaps a college or sports centre would accommodate your proposal?

Networking

Networking and research can be done by various means: attending forums, e.g. nursing, medical, teenage pregnancy; approaching professionals directly, e.g. teenage pregnancy coordinator, family planning service; or contacting local youth organisations, e.g. Connexions (*see* Appendix 1).

Consultation

As well as networking with like-minded professionals, it is vital to consult with young people themselves before setting up a service. Without this we end up setting up what we think young people need rather than what they actually want! Consultation could be in the form of surveys in clinics, schools, colleges or on the street, or a suggestion box in clinics. It is worth noting that surveying in health centres may only generate the opinions of young people who are already confident in accessing services. Peer surveys can be highly effective. Peer surveys recruit from the client group to interview other clients. This is more likely to yield honest discussion as opposed to eliciting what the young person thinks the professional wants to hear. Minority groups identified in the community needs assessment should also be consulted using an appropriate tool. Where are the special needs, religious or ethnic schools and youth groups? Do you need to liaise with community elders to access young people from a particular group? Do you need an advocate to obtain a young person's point of view?

The consultation process should explore young people's opinions on a service. If their views are taken into account regarding the location, timing and environment, it is more likely to be successful as it is tailored to their needs.

The clinic

What is the best location for the project?

Generally young people do not feel comfortable seeking contraceptive and sexual health advice in places where they may meet family and friends. They are also concerned that staff will tell family that they have attended.[1] Therefore, if services are to be provided in a local surgery the best time would be when there are no other clinics, or have the use of a separate waiting room. Other locations could be considered such as schools, colleges and youth centres.

What is the best time?

Daytime services are difficult for young people to attend as they have school, college or work. Late clinics are equally difficult as parents may be wondering where they are. A lunch-time or after school drop-in may be best.

Think carefully about the environment

The clinic environment needs to be welcoming to young people. One study looking at clients' perceptions of a clinic found that most discussion focused on the waiting room rather than the consultation:[2]

> [The waiting room is] too quiet, seems like you're waiting for someone to die ... everyone staring, nothing to do ...
>
> (male aged 23)

If someone came in nervous or anxious they would go out of their minds having to wait so long without anything to do.

(Female aged 22)

This focus could be because this is where clients spend most of their time when attending the clinic. Walk-in clinics often incur long waiting times: magazines, television and refreshments can alleviate possible frustration. A TV or radio helps to mask any discussion between reception staff and young people, who, although they will not be revealing clinical information, may not want people in the waiting room to hear their name and address.

Confidentiality

Research shows repeatedly that young people are most concerned about the level of confidentiality in sexual health and contraception consultations.

A large percentage of young people still think that professionals are obliged to tell their parents about consultations and that they cannot see a doctor alone until they are 16.[3] All health professionals and administrative staff have a duty of confidentiality to clients and have legal codes of practice where this is outlined (*see* Box 2.1).[4]

Box 2.1   Confidentiality: legal codes of practice[4]

Doctors
The General Medical Council states:

'Patients have a right to expect that information about them will be held in confidence by their doctors. Confidentiality is central to trust between doctors and patients.'

Nurses
The United Kingdom Central Council for Nursing, Midwifery and Health Visiting (UKCC, now the NMC: Nursing and Midwifery Council) states that:

'... the patient or client has a right to believe that ... information given in confidence will only be used for the purposes for which it was given and will not be released to others without their permission.'

Administrative staff/management
AMSPAR (the Association of Medical Secretaries, Practice Managers, Administrators and Receptionists) states that:

'Members will strictly observe and uphold the principles of confidentiality. Anything learned from a patient, a medical practitioner, patients' records or correspondence must never be disclosed to any unauthorised person.'

Confidentiality should be stressed at every opportunity. Posters in the waiting room could outline the clinic's confidentiality policy. It could also be stated in publicity leaflets. At each consultation confidentiality should be explained or reiterated. There should be a clinic/service confidentiality policy. All staff should be aware of this policy. Brook and the Royal Society of General Practitioners (RCGP) have put together a confidentiality tool-kit containing sample confidentiality policies and statements that can be used or adapted.[4] The legal and ethical aspects of confidentiality are discussed in more detail in Chapter 3.

Consultation skills

Young people are happier when they are listened to and staff are non-judgemental. The following comments have been made after a contraception consultation:[2]

> [I] asked for a pregnancy test and the same nurse made me feel stupid. 'You're on the injection, you don't need a pregnancy test' as if to say 'silly girl'.

A positive consultation would take a problem-solving approach in partnership with the young person, rather than a prescriptive one. This is where the professional and the client tackle the problem and arrive at a solution together. A problem-solving approach is outlined later in this chapter. Good communication skills are essential for a successful consultation with young people, to set the young person at ease, for them to feel comfortable to discuss sensitive issues and to be empowered to deal effectively with the problem:[2]

> The nurse made me feel relieved and confident in what I was doing. She gave me a choice of contraceptives I could use. She did not force me to do anything or use anything I did not want to. I found her very helpful, informative, professional.

In any consultation technical and medical jargon should be avoided as it risks alienating the client. Young people are forerunners in creating 'in' language and phrases. Unless you are very confident you are up to date with this language it's best to avoid trying to use it as you risk being perceived as out of date or trying too hard.

Young people lack experience in relationships, use of alcohol, work and life in general. They often feel peer pressure to smoke, drink, have sex, hang out with a certain group and dress a certain way. Many lack communication skills to express ideas effectively and to resolve conflicts. In addition they have to adjust to people's expectations of them as they grow older, often causing insecurity and increased emotional responses. Hormones are constantly changing, affecting moods and emotion. An awareness of all this turmoil, which can influence how the young person communicates, helps the communication process to be successful.

Setting boundaries

In a consultation it is helpful to reassure the young person that they are not required to talk about or reveal anything until they are ready to do so; this way they feel in control of the interaction as they gradually learn to trust you.

Sometimes parents attend with the young person. The young person may be happy with this, however the health professional should be aware that the young person may feel inhibited by the presence of a parent and may even be in an abusive situation. Always give young people the opportunity to talk with you privately. When parents are present, ensure both the young person and the parents have a chance to talk and ask questions. For example, if you must ask a parent a question, you should then turn to the adolescent and ask the same question. (It's a good idea to ask parents questions first to avoid putting the teenager on the spot.)

Listening skills

Listening demonstrates to other people that you value what they have to say, which encourages healthy communication. The most common complaint that teenagers have is adults do not listen. This is a quote from a girl's experience of a contraceptive clinic consultation:[2]

> [The nurse] tried to persuade me that my ideas weren't good. I didn't feel listened to or taken seriously ...

Tolerating silence without prompting or idly chatting is also important, giving the young person time to collect their thoughts, reflect on their feelings and decide how much they're willing to share. Listening skills include body language and non-verbal cues. They are intended to encourage the other person to open up and begin to verbalise ideas or feelings freely.

Positive non-verbal cues include the following:

- eye contact
- body relaxed with a forward tilt
- occasional head nod
- a comfortable body distance from the other person.

Verbal cues are tools to make it easy for the other person to talk. They include the following:

- Don't give advice, or ask judgemental questions.
- Use verbal cues such as 'uhmm' and 'I see'.
- Use open-ended questions. (Examples: 'Tell me more' or 'How did that make you feel?')
- Summarising effectively checks your understanding of the person's feelings and situation.
- Keep questions simple.
- Ask relevant questions to clarify facts.

It helps to remember the following:

- Listen for ideas and facts.
- Judge content, not delivery.

- Don't jump to conclusions.
- Keep an open mind.

Problem solving

After having listened to the young person a problem-solving approach is useful. Problem solving is a process in which a person follows a sequence of steps to select a solution from two or more possible choices. Different individuals may face the same situation and select a different solution because of their personal values and goals.

The following is a step-by-step guide to problem solving:

- Clarify the problem – you both must have a clear understanding of the problem.
- Rephrase what you think the young person is saying until both of you agree on the problem.
- If there is more than one problem, discuss which is most important for the young person.
- Explore options to the problem. You may give suggestions and information, but do not give your opinion as to which option you prefer. Let the responsibility of the choice rest with the young person.
- Explore the positive and negative consequences of each choice.
- Draw upon the young person's experience; is he/she able to take a similar experience and apply it to this one. What worked and what did not?
- Let the young person select an option.
- There should be a back-up plan if relevant.
- Have the young person re-attend at an appropriate interval to evaluate the plan.
- If the original plan is not working, restart the problem-solving process.

Outreach

Reaching young people

According to the Durex Report 1999, young people rate general practitioners (GPs) as the most popular regular source for sexual health and contraceptive advice, closely followed by family planning (FP) clinics (*see* Table 2.1).[5] However, friends and schools are the most popular first sources of sexual health information. These are not always the best sources as information from friends can be inaccurate and the level of sex and relationship teaching in schools varies greatly. Parents feature lower down, as do leaflets, TV and magazines. Hence whilst clinics are a recognised source of information there is work to be done to increase the rate of young people accessing a professional service as the first and regular source of information. There is also a need to work with parents to improve communication between parents and young people regarding sexual health.

Friends

The Durex Report illustrates striking facts about where young people access sexual health and contraceptive advice. As mentioned above, for many young

Table 2.1   Durex Report 1999: sources of contraceptive advice[5]

	Regular source %	First source %
Doctor	53	23
FP clinic	24	15
Friends	13	30
Parents	5	15
Magazines/newspapers	15	12
Books	13	13
Brothers/sisters	2	5
Leaflets	12	9
Pharmacists	5	2
Radio	1	1
Sexual partner	12	8
Taught at school	14	31
TV	11	8

people friends are the first source of sexual health and contraceptive information. However, this information may not always be correct. Yet the influence of friends can be positive. One study, asking where new attendees at a clinic had heard about the service, showed the main source to be friends. Almost half of the respondents reported visiting the clinic for the first time with a friend, usually someone already familiar with the service. Friends helped new clients find the clinic and explained its procedures:[2]

> [I] first heard about the clinic through two school friends … [It's] my first visit today, I came in with two school friends after school.
> (Female aged 15)

Relying on friends for support meant new clients often used services close to their friend's house or school rather then their own:[2]

> I am no longer local but I still use the clinic as it's familiar and not frightening to come here.
> (Female aged 23)

Word of mouth is the best publicity for a service; if a young person has a positive experience at a clinic they will tell their friends.

School

The Durex Report showed that an equally important source of sexual health information is school. Other research suggests that both pupils and parents see school as the most appropriate place for sexual health education.[6] Whilst biological aspects of the curriculum can be looked at in science classes, relationship issues, self-esteem and negotiation skills are usually part of the Personal and Social Education (PSE) classes and come under the title of 'Sex and Relationships Education' (SRE). (Work in this area is discussed in Chapter 10.) There is not a set curriculum for PSE and the content of classes can depend on the teacher. PSE is frequently a teacher's second subject. Teaching staff can feel unsure and ill-equipped to teach SRE. Health professionals can support teachers by offering workshops in schools, clinic tours and resources. When health professionals are invited to a school for talks or workshops, it enables young people to discuss issues they may not want to discuss in front of their teachers and introduces them to the health professionals they will see in community clinics. This helps to dispel any fears and preconceived ideas they may have had about the clinics.

Outreach

School is the most obvious place to reach young people; however, it can be beneficial to work with young people in a more informal setting where they feel more in control of events. Outreach work can take place in many settings from youth clubs to fast-food outlets and can range from handing out leaflets and informal chat to planned workshops.

The outreach facilitator should be approachable with an accepting attitude. The young person should be made to feel comfortable to get involved and ask questions. If the individuals carrying out the outreach are those that staff the clinics there is continuity between the services and a familiar face for the young people when they attend.

For workshops, active learning methods are vital. This way young people use analytical thought to come to their own conclusions and are more likely to retain information. (*See* Chapter 10 for more information on outreach work.)

Parents

According to the Durex Report, young people in England rarely go to their parents for sexual health or contraceptive information. Yet good communication with parents/carers regarding sex and contraception is one of the characteristics of countries that have a low teen pregnancy rate.[6] Young people are more likely to delay sexual activity and protect themselves if they have had open and honest discussion with parents and carers from an early age.[7] However, parents don't always feel they have the skills or confidence to raise these issues with their children. Work with parents to increase their confidence in talking to their children about sex and suggest possible resources for the home is an important part of sexual health promotion outreach.

An ideal way to make contact with parents is through school. Contact via an established institution gives credibility to your service. It is generally recognised that schools provide some form of sexual health education. The first task would be to liaise with teaching staff to inform parents of the contents of the SRE classes. Improved liaison between home and school ensures there is continuity and consistency in information and support for the young people.

The aim of a group working with parents would be to build their confidence to have open discussions with their children and thereby increase their children's

---

Box 2.2 'Parent Power': a sex and relationships course for parents and carers of adolescents

'Parent Power' offers a structured course of several evening meetings for parents and carers of young adolescents. It is designed to build self-confidence in communicating with sons and daughters about sexual development and feelings.

Courses are offered to schools who invite parents of one year or tutor group to attend.

The course:

- gives information about puberty
- examines influences, e.g. media, TV, teen magazines
- looks at parents' own attitudes
- explores communicating in the family and the importance of listening to and answering children's questions.

---

knowledge of sexual and reproductive health. The group should focus on increasing parents' sexual health knowledge so they can give accurate information as well as improving communication skills to enable them to communicate effectively with their children. 'Parent Power', a series of sessions offered by East Sussex County Council/Brighton and Hove Personal, Social and Health Education (PSHE) Advisory Team, is an example of successful engagement with parents (*see* Box 2.2).[6]

Engaging parents can be difficult. Little work with parents happens in secondary schools, probably due to the fact that in secondary schools parents tend to have less contact with the school. When groups like this are set up it is often parents who are already talking with their children who are likely to attend. It is also difficult to recruit fathers. Parents need to be proactively and creatively recruited, i.e. through existing parent groups, parent evenings, etc.

Here are two examples of creative work with parents:

Parents from faith groups (often the groups that withdraw their children from SRE classes) can be difficult to engage. A south London group overcame this by liaising with the faith leader. The faith leader nominated certain members of the congregation to attend the sessions. Parents felt honoured to have been chosen by their faith leader to be involved in the project.[6]

A Sheffield group found involving parents as peer educators to speak with other parents about issues to do with sex and sexuality provided them with a positive role model. Parents are trained to run sex education sessions for other parents in community settings (full description in Chapter 10).[6]

Creative use of media

To attract young people to a service the publicity needs to be concise, understandable and contemporary. Research has shown that young people want health publicity to be of a similar standard to commercial publicity:[8]

> It doesn't matter, it could have all the information in the world on it but you're not going to read it 'cause it's so boring ... Yeah, you need something short and to the point.

Credit card health information and club-style flyers have been recent examples of contemporary media used by health services. Paper publicity is not always effective as young people may prefer not to have evidence of where they have been for others to find. Other ways of communicating health promotion messages need to be explored. A good example is the company that makes Evra®, the contraceptive patch, who use text messaging to remind young people when they are due to change a patch. Humour is always a good way of communicating a message:[8]

> Sex is generally regarded as very embarrassing. So if you can get people to laugh about it, they're going to be more open about it and read it.

Most young people have a passion for music. The Young African Caribbean Men's Sexual Health Project in Camden and Islington National Health Service (NHS) Trust maximised on this through working in partnership with a media company, Bigga Fish, to produce a CD with tunes focusing on sexual health messages (*see* Box 2.3).[9]

One way to ensure that media for clinics is appealing to young people is to involve them in their design and production. Involving young people in shaping a project gives them ownership. As a result projects are more likely to be contemporary and reflect young people's needs. In addition, involving media professionals leads to a high production standard and is useful work experience for the young people involved.

Box 2.3   Camden and Islington NHS Trust: Young African Caribbean Men's Sexual Health Project[9]

Mix and Tricks Project
This project worked with a local not-for-profit music and media company run by young people called Bigga Fish. It involved the production of a six-track CD with tunes that feature health promotion messages on sexually transmitted infections (STIs), drugs and relationship issues. Twelve young people were trained in performance and two of them are now working for a professional organisation. They were also trained in writing song lyrics and dance. The project raised awareness around STIs, substance misuse and condom use. It was distributed free to young people at youth clubs, raves and events organised by Bigga Fish.

Minority groups should be considered when designing media for a service. Do media need to be produced in other languages? Could the information be produced pictorially? (This would be useful for young people with learning difficulties as well as those with minority first languages.) Involving young people from these groups in publicity production will ensure that it is effective and appropriate.

Summary

The teenage years are often parodied as a time when reasonable communication is difficult. Yet it is a time when health promotion messages are vital. To effectively communicate with teens involves examining the whole shape of a service, not simply the face-to-face contact. A needs assessment that includes consultation with young people will ensure that the service is appropriate to their needs. The location, timing and publicity of clinics and staff consultation skills should communicate a welcoming message to young people. Creativity in how health promotion messages are being communicated through different media ensures health messages remain fresh and relevant. Research shows that young people would like to receive sexual health information from their parents and from schools, yet lack of support and resources can prevent positive sexual health messages being communicated. Outreach work by sexual health experts with schools and parents can increase teachers' and parents' confidence in dealing with a sensitive subject.

References

1 Tilsley L (1997) Sexual health and teenagers. *Practice Nurse.* 23 May: 541–4.
2 Baraitser P, Blake G, Brown KC *et al.* (2003) Barriers to the involvement of clients in family planning service development: lessons learnt from experience. *Journal of Family Planning and Reproductive Health Care.* **29** (4): 199–203.
3 Davies L (2003) Access by the unaccompanied under-16-year-old adolescent to general practice without parental consent. *Journal of Family Planning and Reproductive Health Care.* **29** (4): 205–7.
4 Royal College of General Practitioners and Brook (2000) *Confidentiality and Young People: improving teenagers' uptake of sexual and other health advice. A toolkit for general practice, primary care groups and trusts.* RCGP, London.
5 The Durex Report (1999) *Spotlight on Sex and Sexual Attitudes in 90's Britain.* Brisbourne LRC Products Ltd, Manchester.
6 Social Exclusion Unit (1999) *Teenage Pregnancy Strategy.* HMSO, London.
7 Mims B and Biordi DL (2001) Communication patterns in African-American families with adolescent mothers of single or repeat pregnancies. *Journal of National Black Nurses Association.* **12** (1): 34–41.
8 Pearson S (2003) Promoting sexual health services to young men: findings from focus group discussions. *Journal of Family Planning and Reproductive Health Care.* **29** (4): 194–8.
9 Teen Pregnancy Conference (2002) Unpublished.

Resources
Needs assessment

- www.hda-online.org.uk/html/resources/publications.asp
  Needs assessment workbook by the Health Development Agency.

- www.show.scot.nhs.uk/nhsfv/fvhealthpromotion/sexualhealth/needsassessment.htm
  An example of a needs assessment by Forth Valley Health Board Health Promotion Department who commissioned the Scottish Council for Research in Education to undertake a sexual health needs analysis of vulnerable young people aged between 14 and 16 who lived in the Forth Valley area.

Communication skills

- Northouse L and Northouse P (1977) *Health Communication: strategies for health professionals.* Appleton and Lange, New York.

- Nolan E, Arnold P, Underman K *et al.* (1999) *Interpersonal Relationships: professional communication skills for nurses.* Saunders, Los Angeles.

- van Servellen G (1996) *Communication Skills for the Healthcare Professional: concepts and techniques.* Aspen Publishers, Maryland.

Working with parents

- *How Much, How Soon?*
  A video that aims to encourage and assist teachers, particularly those new to SRE, to tackle what can be a challenging subject. The video shows SRE being delivered in the classroom together with interviews with education experts, teachers and parents. An accompanying booklet provides useful information on topics covered in the video, including language, teaching techniques and working with parents.
  Available from the Family Planning Association (fpa) direct: PO Box 1078, East Oxford DO, Oxford OX4 6JE. Tel: 01865 719418. www.fpa.org.uk/about/pubs

- Scott L (1996) *Partnership with Parents in Sex Education: a guide for schools and those working with them.* National Children's Bureau, London. www.ncb-books.org.uk/NCB_Books_Sex_Education_16.html

- Hayman S (1998) *You Just Don't Listen: a parent's guide to improving communication with young people.* Vermilion, London.

- Chalke S (1999) *The Parent Talk Guide to the Teenage Years.* Hodder and Stoughton, London.

Working in partnership with young people

- www.teenwise.co.uk
  This website outlines projects run by Teenwise, an organisation that aims to contribute to the reduction of unwanted teenage pregnancy and the improvement of sexual health and other related health and lifestyle outcomes of young people through innovative means of working in Staffordshire. The work is innovative in that it strives to develop partnerships between young people and professionals and between professionals from all sectors. The work will also make use of new technology and exploit more informal educational settings.

CHAPTER 3

Legal issues

This chapter looks at ethical and legal issues surrounding the sexual health of young people. It will examine the issue of consent; its definition, the debate surrounding the age of consent and what the law says on underage consensual sexual intercourse. For professionals working with young people in the area of sexual health child protection considerations are paramount. Sexual abuse is defined and placed in a legal context. Child protection policy and procedure are summarised and the dilemma between maintaining confidentiality and child protection is examined.

Consent

Consent is an agreement to an examination or treatment. Whether a young person is competent to consent to treatment causes many dilemmas for professionals involved in their care. If the child is under 18, and legally a minor, the parent is, in theory, responsible for the young person and should be involved in any decision. The legal age for a sexual relationship is 16 so any young person under 16 engaging in sexual intercourse is acting illegally. Yet, as discussed in the first chapter, a young person doesn't automatically become competent to make reasoned decisions on their 16th birthday. Acquisition of the ability to understand the consequences of a course of action is a gradual process and can begin well before the age of 16. The law does acknowledge this. It is recognised that children and young people have rights regarding what happens to their bodies and can have the ability to make a reasoned and rational decision.

Young people under 16 are legally able to consent to or refuse treatment provided the health professional has assessed their understanding of the procedure and any possible consequences. The Human Rights Act 1998[1] and the United Nations (UN) Convention on the Rights of the Child,[2] to which the UK is a signatory, states that the wishes of a young person must be taken into account when considering their best interests. The Children Act 1989 gave children the authority to consent to and refuse treatment.[3]

Within England the legal age for heterosexual and homosexual intercourse is 16 years. However, although not legal, children between the ages of 13 and 15 are considered able to consent to sexual intercourse. Children below the age of 13 are deemed legally incompetent to consent to sexual activity and as such all sexual intercourse would be considered non-consensual.[4]

There was some confusion in the early 1980s regarding the issuing of contraceptives to girls under 16 and whether their parents should be involved. In 1974, the Department of Health and Social Security (DHSS) issued a memo of guidance to doctors advising that contraceptive advice could be given to girls aged under 16 without informing their parents and that they should always ask the girl's permission to tell her parents. However, the memo was followed up in 1980 by an adage: the need to persuade the girl to involve the parents or guardian and that the decision to involve the parents or not lay with the clinician. Naturally the way this was interpreted varied widely between clinicians. Some carried on as before, advising and issuing contraception to under 16s and encouraging the young woman to talk to her parents; others were told they would have to bring their parents to the appointment. As a result young people felt that confidential advice and treatment were not available to under-16s.[5]

Eventually, following one mother's unsuccessful attempt to gain assurance that her daughters would not be provided with contraceptive advice or treatment without her consent, clearer and more explicit guidelines were produced. These guidelines made clear that health professionals could provide contraceptive advice and treatment to young people provided that certain conditions were met. These conditions are called the Fraser Guidelines,[6] named after the judge who presided over the case. Each time a young person consults for treatment, an assessment should be made of their competence to consent.

This judgement referred specifically to doctors but it is considered to apply to other health professionals working with young people. It may also be interpreted as covering youth workers and health promotion workers who may be giving contraceptive advice and condoms to young people under 16, but this has not been tested in court.

The Fraser Guidelines

Health professionals are able to provide contraceptive advice and treatment to under-16s as long as the following conditions are met:

- the young person understands the professional's advice
- the young person is encouraged to inform their parents
- the young person is likely to begin, or to continue having, sexual intercourse with or without contraceptive treatment
- unless the young person receives contraceptive treatment, their physical or mental health, or both, are likely to suffer
- the young person's best interests require them to receive contraceptive advice or treatment with or without parental consent.

Although these criteria specifically refer to contraception, the principles are deemed to apply to other treatments, including abortion.

NB. Similar provision is made in Scotland by The Age of Legal Capacity (Scotland) Act 1991. In Northern Ireland, although separate legislation applies, the then Department of Health and Social Services Northern Ireland stated that there was no reason to suppose that the House of Lords' decision would not be followed by the Northern Ireland Courts.

Consent and young people with learning disabilities

Young people with learning disabilities should have the same access to services as other young people. However, their learning difficulty may make it hard to obtain consent through routine proformas. Professionals working with this group need to be creative when presenting information to young people with learning difficulties so they can understand their options and the consequences of choices to the best of their ability. This may involve presenting the information pictorially, using other forms of communication aids, e.g. Makaton,* or an advocate. More discussion regarding supporting young people with learning difficulties is found in Chapter 8.

Access to health services by under-16s

Despite the Fraser Guidelines being in existence for nearly 20 years there are still health professionals who will not see an unaccompanied child under 16 years of age. One research study showed that 91% of professionals in general practice would agree to consult with an unaccompanied under 16-year-old, leaving 9% who wouldn't, and 15% of GPs and practice nurses were not comfortable implementing the Fraser Guidelines.[7] Although these are by far the minority, it can lead to young people not being able to access the services and advice they require. Every effort should be made to communicate to health professionals the legal rights of the child to advice and treatment as well as to inform young people of their rights.

Age of consent debate

Debate surrounding the age of consent presents extreme viewpoints. Some feel that the age should be lowered to reflect current sexual activity of young people; some feel that it is fine as it is, reflecting an age between childhood and adulthood; some that it should be raised to protect young people from unwanted pregnancy and STIs; and some that it should be abolished so that sexuality and sex is de-criminalised.

Proposed changes in the law regarding the age of consent and sexual activity will criminalise any sexual activity under the age of 16.[8] This has raised the debate over whether 16 is an appropriate age for consent to sexual intercourse. The Channel 4 television programme *Sex Before 16: where the law is failing* presented a comprehensive debate on the age of consent. The programme was supplemented by information on the internet.[9] The opinions amongst the young people they interviewed varied:

> There's no point in having an age – people do what they want to do. If they want to have sex, they will have sex.

> Should be raised to 18 ... [There are] too many young parents and they don't know what to do in that situation.

---

* A sign and symbol language programme for teaching communication, language and literacy skills to children and adults with communication and learning difficulties.

It's right how it is – halfway between your adult- and childhood.

Twelve is a good age to have sex.

Sixteen is good, it's a necessary guideline.

Box 3.1   Channel 4 age of consent vote[9]

There were 3366 votes on what should happen to the age of consent in the UK following the Channel 4 programme *Sex Before 16: where the law is failing*:

- 34% thought the age of consent should be reduced to 14
- 35% thought it should stay at 16
- 13% thought it should be raised to 18
- 18% thought it should be abolished.

An online vote after the programme further illustrated the mixed opinion amongst young people (*see* Box 3.1).

There is currently no age of consent for boys having heterosexual sex. The age of consent refers to the age of the girl. The 2003 Sexual Offences Reform Bill[8] proposes to extend the current age of consent laws so that all sexual acts, not just penetrative sex, will become a criminal offence if at least one of the people involved is under 16. The main concern in the minds of policy makers is to protect young people from abuse by people older than themselves. This is, of course, a very important consideration, however the bill will by default criminalise people under the age of 16 for consensual sexual acts with other people of similar age.

What are the origins of the current law on the age of consent? Campaigners in the 1860s, when the age of consent stood at 12, fought to stop young girls being sold to brothels. They succeeded in getting Parliament to raise the age to 13. This was then raised to 16 in 1885 when an account was published in a journal of how easy it was to purchase a 13-year-old for prostitution. The concern now is whether the current age of consent at 16 is still reasonable for young people.

Many young people are already having sexual experiences long before the legal age of consent. One viewpoint is that the law needs to recognise this to be able to give the proper advice and support to prevent diseases, unwanted pregnancies and abuse. If 14-year-olds are not legally allowed to have sex, it is very difficult to openly discuss it with them. On the whole, young people do not pay any heed to the law when contemplating sexual relations:[9]

If you feel the time is right ... I don't think anyone should be stopped.

It's nature – you can't have a law against nature.

The law isn't relevant to me. When I've found someone and I'm confident to lose my virginity, I'm not going to think about the law.

Bliss, a magazine for girls (readership is females aged 12–17), conducted a survey regarding girls' sexual experiences. A third had already had sexual intercourse; the majority of those who had had sex were under 16, and a significant proportion under 12 (*see* Box 3.2).[9]

Box 3.2 *Bliss* **survey 2003: girls' sexual experiences**[9]

- 32% of readers have already had sex (readership 12–17)
- 39% had done more than kissing
- 83% of those who had had sexual intercourse were under 16
- 12% were under 12

On the other hand, critics argue that today's culture is becoming increasingly sex obsessed – through adverts, TV and provocative clothing – and this is pressurising teenagers to try to keep up with what they perceive to be the correct way to behave by being sexually promiscuous. Lowering the age of consent is sending yet another message that young people are expected to have sex early.

Opponents of change believe that lowering the age of sexual consent will in fact encourage young people to have sex earlier and place them at greater risk of diseases, unwanted pregnancies and abuse. However, this is not necessarily the case. Some countries have a lower age of consent and a higher age of first intercourse. For example, in Spain the age of consent is 13 and age of first sex is 19 for girls and 18 for boys; in Los Angeles in America the age of consent is 18 and age of first sex is 17; and in Chile the age of consent is 12 and age of first sex is 15 for girls and 14 for boys.[9] We would need to examine to what extent the culture in each country influences sexual behaviour and how it could be compared to Great Britain.

In addition, apparent recent increases in teen sexual activity do not necessarily mean that any more people are having sex earlier than in previous generations. These days we are more honest and efficient at recording data and society has a more open attitude to young people's sexuality.

However, if sexual activity under 16 is criminalised it will mean that young people will receive the message that they are doing something wrong and will not feel confident to seek sexual health and contraceptive advice. As it stands at the moment it could be said that the law is hypocritical, setting the age of consent at 16 yet making contraception available to under-16s to ensure young people break the law safely! One way to deal with this reality, and to continue current positive trends (such as a decline in unwanted teenage pregnancies), is to legally recognise that teenagers are having sex at a younger age; young people will then feel free to seek advice, counselling and direction in their relationships.

Setting an age of consent is considered by some as arbitrary; a young person may be physically mature but not necessarily emotionally ready for a sexual relationship. An age of consent is a barrier that, if removed, gives young people freedom to talk, seek advice and take responsibility for their own actions.

One proposal would be to set the age of consent at the border between childhood and adolescence, and not between adolescence and adulthood. This would maintain childhood innocence whilst supporting consensual teenage experimentation. Interestingly, no country has an age of consent lower than 12; nor has any country abolished the age of consent.

Whatever the conclusion, it is essential that the focus should shift towards education and communication to support young people in making informed choices rather than legislation that criminalises sexual activity.

Abuse

Child sexual abuse is the sexual molestation of children by adults or older children ('sexual' here means any activity that leads to sexual arousal in the perpetrator). The Government paper *Working Together to Safeguard Children* describes it as:[10]

> ... forcing or enticing a child or young person to take part in sexual activities, whether or not the child is aware of what is happening. The activities may include penetrative (e.g. rape or buggery) or non-penetrative acts. They may include non-contact activities, such as involving children in looking at pornographic material or watching sexual activities, or encouraging children to behave in sexually inappropriate ways.

This document is described in more detail later in the chapter.

It is estimated that at least one in four males and one in three females will have encountered some form of sexual abuse before reaching the age of 18.[11] The National Society for the Prevention of Cruelty to Children's (NSPCC) study *Child Maltreatment* found that, contrary to stereotype, sexual abuse by a parent or care-giver is relatively rare and that sexual abuse by a relative most commonly involves a brother or stepbrother. However, a more frequent perpetrator than a relative is someone known to but unrelated to the child. The most common age to suffer abuse by a known but unrelated perpetrator is between 13 and 15; most of the victims are girls (*see* Box 3.3).[12] Very few victims told anyone at the time; if they did they were most likely to have confided in a friend, sometimes in a relative, and, rarely, in a professional.[13]

As well as being traumatic for the young person at the time, the abuse can have psychological consequences in later life such as depression and anxiety, and lead to self-harm and even suicide.[11] Many of those abused never report the abuse: 15% of a national sample of 998 children aged 8–11 years said they would not talk to someone if they were experiencing sexual abuse.[14]

Children who are abused sexually are often groomed and trained, the process occurring over months or years. Children may develop a pattern of adjustment to the abuse, displaying characteristics such as secrecy, helplessness, self-blame, delayed disclosure and retraction.[15]

Box 3.3   Summary of the NSPCC *Child Maltreatment* study[12]

A total of 2869 18–24 year-olds were asked about their childhood experiences:

- 1% had suffered sexual abuse by a parent
- 3% had suffered sexual abuse by another family member (most commonly brother or stepbrother)
- 11% had suffered a sexual experience against their wishes by another unrelated but known person.

Sexual Offences Act 2003

The Sexual Offences Act 2003 for England and Wales[16] states that it is an offence for a man or boy aged 10 or over to have sexual intercourse with a young woman aged 13, 14 or 15. However, this is qualified by the defence that:

- the man or boy believes himself to be validly married to the young woman (even if this is not the case), or
- he is 23 or under at the time of the offence, has not previously been charged with an offence of this kind and believes the young woman to be 16 or over.

It is an absolute offence for a man or boy aged 10 or over to have intercourse with a girl aged 12 or under. There can be no defence in such a case.

Sexual exploitation, such as involvement in prostitution, remains a child protection issue until the young person reaches the age of 18 years.

Once an adult or child has been convicted or cautioned in relation to an offence against a child they are classified and become known as 'Schedule 1 Offenders'. The Act requires certain categories of sex offenders to notify the police of their current whereabouts. In this way, agencies with child protection responsibilities are able to manage and monitor the risks offenders present to children.

Homosexuality

The same Act legalised homosexual acts between men provided that they are both 16 or over in England, Wales and Scotland, 17 or over in Northern Ireland, and the act takes place in private.

The only offence related to lesbianism is that of indecent assault. Provided both women consent, and neither is under the age of consent, acts of lesbianism are legal.

Child protection

The Children Act 1989[3] sets out the legal requirements for child protection practice. It outlines clear policy regarding child protection issues, and referral pathways to support professionals in often complicated and difficult situations. Box 3.4 summarises the Children Act.

Ten years after the Children Act the Government published a national strategy for child protection practice. Entitled *Working Together to Safeguard Children*, this document outlines how all agencies and professionals should work together to promote children's welfare and protect them from abuse and neglect.[10] It states that each health authority must appoint a designated nurse and doctor to take the strategic lead in all aspects of the health service contribution to safeguarding children. The primary care trust has the responsibility for child protection services across all health providers. These named health professionals are the point of contact within the health service for child protection advice.

Box 3.4 Summary of the Children Act 1989[3]

Purpose
- The Children Act 1989 is based on the belief that children are generally best looked after within the family, with both parents playing a full part and without resort to legal proceedings.
- The welfare of the child is the paramount consideration.
- Courts will not make orders regarding children unless the parents are in disagreement about where they should live, what sort of contact they should maintain etc., or if there are concerns about their welfare (different types of court order are listed).
- Children should always be consulted (subject to age and understanding) and kept informed about what will happen to them. Court decisions about their future upbringing should be responsive to their needs. Parents and the children's wider family circle should continue to have a role to play in the lives of their children even when they are living apart.
- Children's issues must be determined as soon as possible so that minimum disruption is caused to the child's life. To minimise delay, the court must draw up a timetable in respect of subsequent proceedings.

Statutory check-list
The court must have regard to:

- the wishes and feelings of the child concerned
- their physical, emotional and educational needs
- the likely effect of any changes in their circumstances
- their age, sex, background and any characteristics which the court considers relevant
- any harm which they have suffered or are at risk of suffering
- how capable their parents are, or other significant adult is, of meeting their needs
- the range of powers available to the court.

Local procedures

Local Area Child Protection Committees (ACPCs) were established following the Children Act 1989, whose aim is to coordinate and promote effective inter-agency work. Every local authority is required to have an ACPC, made up of all agencies with responsibility for services to children. Social services (the lead agency), health, education, police, probation and the voluntary sector are all represented. The ACPC is informed by the document *Working Together to Safeguard Children*.[10] The main points of the document are:

- to promote support to families under stress
- to consider the wider needs of the child and family

- to focus on the welfare and safety of the child
- to outline the different types of abuse and neglect
- to support skilled assessment by professionals working with children
- to recognise adult and children's services have complementary roles and need to work together
- to set out the roles and responsibilities of ACPCs, and ways of working
- to provide guidance on the steps that should be followed if there are concerns about the welfare of a child
- to outline the role and importance of inter-agency training
- to outline particular considerations which apply to safeguarding children in a range of specific circumstances:

  - children living away from home
  - responding to allegations of abuse made against professionals, foster carers and volunteers; whether as individuals or in organised or multiple abuse contexts, including historical abuse
  - vulnerability of disabled children
  - guidance on abuse by children and young people
  - relationship between domestic violence and harm to children
  - material on children involved in prostitution.

The document also contains the *Framework for the Assessment of Children in Need and Their Families*.[17] This framework provides a systematic basis for collecting and analysing information to support professional judgements on the best interests of the child. The intention is that practitioners use the framework to gain an understanding of a child's developmental needs, the capacity of parents or care-givers to respond appropriately to those needs and the impact of wider family and environmental factors on the parents and child (*see* Appendix 2).

Confidentiality

Confidentiality is where information shared between professional and client remains within the consultation. Everyone is entitled to a confidential consultation, regardless of age. This can only be broken if there are child protection or safety concerns for the client or others. Concern regarding confidentiality is often quoted by young people when asked about barriers to seeking sexual health advice.[18] Conversely, professionals are concerned that if there are child protection issues they cannot guarantee complete confidentiality.

Young people under the age of 16 have the same right to confidentiality as any other patient. If someone under 16 is not judged mature enough to consent to treatment (*see* Fraser Guidelines, p. 34), the consultation itself can still remain confidential. Professionals working with young people have a duty of confidentiality. They must not disclose anything learned from a person who has consulted or whom they have examined or treated, without that person's agreement. Confidentiality may only be broken in the most exceptional circumstances where the health, safety or welfare of the client, or others, would be at grave risk.

Providing confidential sexual health services to young people can raise concerns amongst professionals regarding sexual activity and the law. While young people are entitled to the same degree of confidentiality as adults and can consent to examination and treatment if judged to be Fraser-competent, their sexual activity may be unlawful either due to their age, the age of their partner or if they are involved in prostitution. Sexual activity is a particular issue for the under-13s; they can be judged Fraser-competent to consent to examination and treatment but are regarded as incapable of consenting to sexual activity, requiring referral to child protection services or the police if they are sexually active.

Although every effort is made to give young people equal rights to confidentiality there are certain occasions when a professional may have to consider disclosure of information to child protection services:[19]

- where a child is sexually active under the age of 13
- where a child between the ages of 13 and 15 is having consensual sex with a partner who is 24 years or over
- where there is disclosure of or suspected sexual abuse
- where the disclosure of information may be the only way to protect the client from serious harm
- where other children may potentially be at risk
- children under 18 who are involved in commercial sex work.

These situations are examples of clinical situations where disclosure will need to be considered. Naturally, a balance needs to be found between the need to protect the child from harm and the child's right to confidentiality. The aim is to develop a relationship of trust with the young person. Each situation must be assessed individually before any decision to disclose is made. Information is shared with other professionals on a need-to-know basis.

If the young person is opposed to the requirement to break confidentiality, attempts should be made to work with them to make consent to disclosure acceptable. It may be possible to work with the young person over a period of time in order to obtain consent, unless there is evidence of immediate danger or risk to another child.

Clinicians providing these services have to weigh up the child protection issues for these young people, while considering their needs and rights to confidential care. If a service is not seen to be confidential there is a risk that it will not be accessed, or that those attending will not be honest about their age and/or sexual activity, and may not disclose abuse or exploitation. This can have serious health implications: abuse might go unrecognised and the opportunity to support the young person and for intervention would be lost.

Teamworking

The contribution of all professionals to the safeguarding of children is essential. Often many professionals come into contact with a young person who is being abused. The young person may confide in a professional or the professional may get a feeling that something is not right. This information or feeling may not seem important on its own; the professional may think it's not significant enough to take further. However, other professionals may be in a similar position and the combination of information can build a picture that will warrant an investigation.

It can be difficult to assess the significance of certain information. Discussion with clinicians reveals that most are comfortable dealing with disclosures of definite abuse. More often, however, they are faced with ambiguous situations. These vary from case to case and should be dealt with on an individual basis. To help identify and clarify the concern, it is helpful to discuss the situation with other members of your team or the named professional with responsibility for child protection issues in the team. Often child protection issues are complicated with layers of concern: the immediate physical safety of the child, the psychological condition of the child (they may not think they are in an abusive situation), protection from STIs and pregnancy, etc.

As discussed earlier, there is a designated nurse and doctor responsible for child protection within community health services. As they are constantly dealing with child protection cases they have the ability to draw out the prime concerns for the young person, and the expertise to advise on a plan of action for the particular situation. It is possible to discuss your concerns without identifying the young person involved.

The social worker is the central point for reporting any concerns you may have regarding a young person. It is possible to ring social services and speak informally to the duty social worker about a situation and take their advice on whether the concern should be formally reported. The duty social worker will ask you for the name and address of the child; this is to see if they already have a file on the child or other children in the family. This is part of a social worker's role – to collect information and build a picture of what is happening in a family or situation.

Record keeping

At every step it is essential to record your concerns and actions taken. Records should include objective observations, the content of discussion between you and the young person, discussions with other professionals, and times and dates of contact. These notes should be written at the time of contact or very soon afterwards to ensure accuracy of information. The notes should follow the child if they move so professionals who will be coming into contact with the young person will have information regarding their situation and can carry on any work started.

Summary

The issue of consent can cause concerns for the professional working with young people. The Children Act and Fraser Guidelines provide specific guidance regarding sexual activity and young people, although the age of consent remains a contentious issue. Where there are child protection concerns there are clear procedures to follow through the ACPC. Child protection issues may not always be clear cut; in this instance professionals may consult with social services or the named health professionals for child protection while respecting a young person's right to confidentiality.

Professionals are also supported through Government guidance in the paper *Working Together to Safeguard Children*[10] and its accompanying *Framework for the Assessment of Children in Need and Their Families.*[17]

References

1   Cabinet Office (1998) *The Human Rights Act*. HMSO, London.
2   UN General Assembly (1989) *United Nations Convention on the Rights of the Child*. United Nations, New York.
3   Cabinet Office (1989) *The Children Act 1989*. HMSO, London.
4   British Medical Association (2000) *Consent, Rights and Choices in Health Care for Children and Young People*. BMA, London.
5   Sutherland C (2001) *Women's Health: a handbook for nurses*. Churchill Livingstone, London.
6   Gillick *v* West Norfolk and Wisbech Area Health Authority (1985) 1 AC 12, 184 G.
7   Davies L (2003) Access by the unaccompanied under 16-year-old adolescent to general practice without parental consent. *Journal of Family Planning and Reproductive Health Care*. **29** (4): 205–7.
8   Cabinet Office (2003) *Sexual Offences Reform Bill*. HMSO, London.
9   www.channel4.com/health/microsites/A/adultat14/consent/aoc_consent.shtml (2003)
10 Department of Health (1999) *Working Together to Safeguard Children: a guide to inter-agency working to safeguard and promote the welfare of children*. HMSO, London.
11 National Society for the Prevention of Cruelty to Children (1997) *Childhood Matters: commission of inquiry into the prevention of child abuse*. NSPCC, Leicester.
12 National Society for the Prevention of Cruelty to Children (2000) *Child Maltreatment in the United Kingdom: a study of the prevalence of child abuse and neglect*. NSPCC, Leicester.
13 Bastable R (2003) The sexually abused child. *The Practitioner*. **247**: 934–9.
14 National Society for the Prevention of Cruelty to Children (1997) *Talking About My Generation*. NSPCC, Leicester.
15 Barker J and Hodes D (2002) *The Child in Mind: a child protection handbook*. City and Hackney Primary Care Trust, London.
16 Cabinet Office (2003) *Sexual Offences Act*. HMSO, London.
17 Department for Education and Employment (2000) *Framework for the Assessment of Children in Need and Their Families*. HMSO, London.
18 Bekaert S (2003) Improving healthcare provision for teenagers. *Practice Nurse*. 28 March: 38–45.
19 General Medical Council (2000) *Confidentiality: protecting and providing information*. GMC, London.

Resources
Child protection

- Barker J and Hodes D (2002) *The Child in Mind: a child protection handbook*. City and Hackney Primary Care Trust, London. Handbook showing how best to work with vulnerable children. Designed to complement the national strategy for child protection (*Working Together to Safeguard Children*) and the local ACPC procedures.

Available from City and Hackney Primary Care Trust. Tel: 020 7683 4000. enquiries@chpct.nhs.uk

- Howarth J (2000) *The Child's World: assessing children in need*. NSPCC, Leicester. Training pack accompanying the Department of Health's *Framework for the Assessment of Children in Need and Their Families*.
  Available from the NSPCC National Training Centre, 3 Gilmour Close, Beaumont Leys, Leicester LE4 1EZ. Tel: 0116 234 7200. www.nspcc.org.uk/inform/Training/ChildsWorld. asp

- Carter YH and Bannon MJ (2002) *The Role of Primary Care in the Protection of Children from Abuse and Neglect*. A position paper of the Royal College of General Practitioners, London.
  Available from the Royal College of General Practitioners, 14 Prince's Gate, London SW7 1PU. Tel: 020 7581 3232. info@rcgp.org.uk

- www.rcgp.org.uk/rcgp/corporate/position/childprotection.pdf

- Department of Health (2003) *What to do if you're worried a child is being abused*. www.publications.doh.gov.uk/safeguardingchildren
  Flowchart for referral and summary document.

Confidentiality

- Royal College of General Practitioners and Brook (2000) *Confidentiality and Young People: improving teenagers' uptake of sexual and other health advice. A toolkit for general practice, primary care groups and trusts*. RCGP, London. Resource outlining law and issues surrounding confidentiality, with copiable overheads for teaching and adaptable proformas for use in the clinical setting.
  Available from the Royal College of General Practitioners, 14 Prince's Gate, London SW7 1PU. Tel: 020 7581 3232. info@rcgp.org.uk

- National Deaf Children's Society (1990) *You Choose*. www.ndcs.org.uk/information/ndcs_publications/you_choose.html. Child-friendly book addressing the difficult subject of knowing who to tell about secrets which the child may feel uncomfortable about sharing.

- *Here to listen, not to tell*
  An A3 poster on confidentiality.
  Available from Brook Publications, 421 Highgate Studios, 53–79 Highgate Road, London NW5 1TL. Tel: 020 7284 6056. admin@brookcentres.org.uk

- *Confidentiality: a training manual for staff providing sex advice to young people*
  Available from Brook Publications, 421 Highgate Studios, 53–79 Highgate Road, London NW5 1TL. Tel: 020 7284 6056. admin@brookcentres.org.uk

- *Trust*
  A 10-minute video designed to trigger discussion on confidentiality policy and young people.
  Available from the Royal College of General Practitioners, 14 Prince's Gate, London SW7 1PU. Tel: 020 7581 3232. info@rcgp.org.uk

CHAPTER 4

Teenage pregnancy

Teenage pregnancy is a hot issue and has been identified by the Government as an area that needs particular attention. Thus a specific department, the Teenage Pregnancy Unit, has been set up by the Government to identify and deal with issues pertaining to teen pregnancy. It is commonly thought with the coverage and publicity that teenage pregnancy receives that it is statistically the worst it has ever been in England and Wales. However, while we do not compare favourably with neighbouring European countries (see Table 4.2 overleaf), the statistics have been steadily improving since the 1970s. Teenagers are in fact far less likely to get pregnant today than they were in the early 1970s. The conception rate in 1970 was 82.4 per 1000 15–19 year-olds compared to 43.8 in 2000. Since 1998 the teenage conception rate has declined. The decline in teenage motherhood is even more striking. In 1970, 71.4 per 1000 15–19 year-olds had a baby, almost twice the rate as that for 2000 (see Table 4.1).[1]

These improvements have been ascribed to the increased availability of contraception, the introduction of the Abortion Act in 1967 that increased the availability of legal abortion, and heightened awareness of sexual health and contraceptive issues amongst the population as a whole.

Despite an overall reduction in teen pregnancy in recent decades, England and Wales still do not compare favourably with other Western countries, as Table 4.2 illustrates.[3]

In previous centuries people generally married younger and child bearing was traditionally reserved for marriage. Adolescence is currently associated with being a time for education, and achieving financial and social independence prior to forming relationships (as discussed in Chapter 1). Having children during this time could be seen as interrupting and hindering achievement in these areas, and making it difficult to achieve in the future.

Table 4.1 Teen conception statistics for England, 1998–2001[2]

Year	Total conceptions	Conception rate	Per cent leading to legal abortion
1998	41 089	47.0	42.4
1999	39 247	45.3	43.5
2000	38 690	43.8	44.8
2001	38 439	42.3	46.0

Table 4.2 Teenage birth, abortion and pregnancy rates per year (per 1000 women aged 15–19) per developed country for 2000[3]

Country	Birth rate	Abortion rate	Pregnancy rate
England and Wales	28.4	18.6	47
Australia	19.8	23.8	43.6
Belgium	9.1	5	14.1
Canada	24.2	21.2	45.4
France	10	10.2	20.2
Germany	12.5	3.6	16.1
Italy	6.9	5.1	12
Netherlands	8.2	4	12.2
New Zealand	34	20	54
Russian Federation	45.6	56.1	101.7
Scotland	27.1	14	41.1
Spain	7.8	4.5	12.3
Sweden	7.7	17.2	24.9
United States of America	54.4	29.2	83.6

Young parents find it difficult to finish their education and/or find and hold down a job.[4] This leaves them socially isolated and financially disadvantaged. The Government has labelled this 'social exclusion' and it is this, rather than teenage pregnancy *per se*, that they want to help young people avoid.

Statistics

There are great regional variations in statistics. The teenage conception rate is considerably higher in deprived areas of the country compared with affluent areas. These areas are characterised by poor levels of education and poor job prospects. Teenage pregnancy rates in some of the poorer boroughs of London are far greater than in the rest of the country.[1]

The likelihood of a pregnant teenager having an abortion decreases with age. Of those aged under 14, 59% have abortions; for 15-year-olds the figure is 52%; at 17, 40% and at 19, 35% (figures for England and Wales in 2000).[1] For more details regarding abortion, *see* Appendix 3.

Fewer children have been given for adoption in recent years as a direct result of legalised abortion. In 1975 more than 20 000 children were given for adoption; in 1985 the figure was 7000 and in 1995, 6000. Giving a child for adoption is more likely amongst teens with economic/educational aspirations and from higher socio-economic groups.[2]

It is worth noting that statistics don't make a distinction between planned and unplanned pregnancy in teenage years. This would suggest that organisations collecting and collating these statistics see all teenage pregnancy as a problem. Conversely, some cultures see teenage pregnancy (usually within marriage) as acceptable. Often there is extended family support for the young mother within these traditions and a high level of education or work is not expected or required of mothers. However, these groups are more likely to fall into lower socio-economic groups than the national average.[5]

Government targets

The picture is not all doom and gloom: young people can be responsible in seeking out contraceptive advice and have more choices available to them (e.g. contraceptive clinics and abortion). However, the social exclusion that usually accompanies teenage parenthood is an important issue. Young parents can become trapped in a poverty cycle from which it is difficult to escape.

Social exclusion is a shorthand term for what can happen when people or areas suffer from a combination of linked problems such as unemployment, poor skills, low incomes, poor housing, high-crime environments, bad health and family break-down. The Social Exclusion Unit was set up by the Government to help improve action to reduce social exclusion; this involved several agencies.[6] From this the Teenage Pregnancy Unit was set up to specifically focus on issues surrounding teenage pregnancy.

The Teenage Pregnancy Strategy takes a preventative and educative approach to help young people avoid becoming young parents; and promotes strategies to support teenage parents improve their options in life. Box 4.1 contains a summary of the Teenage Pregnancy Strategy – the full document can be accessed on the Teenage Pregnancy Unit website.[7]

Box 4.1   Teenage Pregnancy Strategy summary[7]

- Teenage pregnancy rates in England are significantly higher than in other European countries.
- Teenage pregnancy affects all areas of the country, although rates are higher in poorer areas.
- Teenage pregnancy rates are higher for vulnerable young people, i.e. those in care, excluded from school, etc.
- Teenage parents are more likely to live in poverty and be unemployed.
- Children of teenage parents have a higher death and accident rate than those of older mothers.

Why are rates so high?
Low expectations
Teenage pregnancy is more common amongst young people who have been disadvantaged in childhood and have poor expectations of education or the job market. Young women see no reason not to get pregnant.

Ignorance
Young people lack accurate knowledge of contraception, STIs, relationships and being a parent.

Mixed messages
Young people are surrounded by sexually explicit material yet adults generally do not talk openly about sex and protection, resulting in unprotected sex.

Two main goals:
* reducing the rate of teenage conceptions, with the specific aim of halving the rate of conceptions among under-18s by 2010
* getting more teenage parents into education, training or employment, to reduce their risk of long-term social exclusion.

Action plan
* *National campaign* – target young people and parents with the facts about teenage pregnancy and parenthood, advice on how to deal with pressures to have sex, importance of using contraception if they do have sex.
* *Joined-up action* – appointment of local coordinators to pull together all the services that have a role in preventing teenage pregnancy or supporting those that become parents.
* *Better prevention* – better education in and out of school, access to contraception, working with parents and targeting at-risk groups, especially young men.
* *Better support* – for pregnant teenagers and teenage parents to return to education.

Consequences of teenage pregnancy[8]

When I told my family about my pregnancy I received mixed feelings from them. My nan was very disappointed in me but I expected that anyway as she is from an older generation. My grandad didn't really say anything. My boyfriend's family were really upset when I told them and they still haven't accepted it now, and my daughter is 18 months old. Friends at school didn't take to it very well. When you're in a group and they're all having sex with guys then it's ok, but as soon as one of you gets pregnant then it's different. None of them came to see me when I was pregnant or afterwards. I didn't want them to anyway as they had ignored me and I was now different to them anyway. It wouldn't be the same for me as I had responsibilities while they were still silly young teenagers.

Education

There is a clear link between education and teenage pregnancy rates. The level of education is inversely proportional to numbers of teenage pregnancies – the higher the level of education the less teen pregnancy.[9] This appears to be for two reasons:

young people who don't see themselves going on in education will not feel they have lost any opportunities by becoming young parents, and once a young person becomes pregnant the chances of them completing their education are greatly reduced. Despite good intentions it can be difficult to combine a highly timetabled school life with a not so timetabled child. It is difficult for schools to be flexible and the struggle to combine motherhood and education can deter young people from continuing their schooling. If teen mothers fail to stay in school there is also a greater likelihood of a closer spaced subsequent birth.[10] Therefore poor academic performance is considered a determinant and consequence of child bearing too early.

Poverty

Nationally, the risk of becoming a teenage mother is almost ten times higher for a girl whose family is in social class V (unskilled manual) than those in social class 1 (professional) (*see* Appendix 4 for all social class definitions).[11] Once a young woman has become a teenage parent, it is difficult to finish education and/or find and hold down a job and establish independence from family and state. This perpetuates the poverty cycle. In addition, research has shown there is an increased chance of becoming a teenage mother if their mother had a teenage pregnancy.[2]

Many teenage mothers have family support. Seven out of ten 15 and 16-year-olds and one half of 17 and 18-year-olds stay in the family home with their child.[2] This has psychological as well as monetary benefits for the young person as she is likely to have help with childcare and be more able to return to school or work. It does, however, put financial pressure on the extended family.

Health

There are negative health consequences for young parents and their children. Pregnant teens often do not seek or get adequate prenatal care, missing out on important scans and blood tests as well as access to support networks.[4] Children of teens are at increased risk of low birth-weight, infant mortality, sudden infant death syndrome, and increased rates of illness and injury.[11]

It is therefore important to support young parents in order to avoid this possible poverty cycle. This can be done through projects that enable young mums to attend school or work and achieve some independence both socially and financially. Specific healthcare provision for young pregnant women, such as teen antenatal clinics and young mothers and fathers groups, can give young parents peer support and self-esteem to tackle the issues they face. One good example is the Young Fathers' Project in Cornwall (*see* Box 4.2).[2]

Box 4.2   Young Fathers' Project[2]

The Young Fathers' Project is a Sure Start (*see* Appendix 5) initiative to support young fathers based in the Penzance and Camborne area of Cornwall.

A development worker has been appointed to take forward work with young fathers. The primary aim is to support young men's relationships with their children and the mother of their child.

There are two groups that meet once a week. The groups act as an informal support group for young fathers who meet with the development worker for a chat, plan trips out with and without their children, and sometimes focus on a specific project. The groups are small – four to five men regularly attend.

Two young fathers have been trained as peer educators as part of the peer education package. They go to schools to speak to 14 and 15-year-old boys about the realities of being a father.

The development worker also undertakes one-to-one support with young fathers. This is used by those who are experiencing problems, such as fathers who have sole care of their children, those who are experiencing problems with their partners, etc.

Influences on young people's choices

There are many influences that impinge on a young person's sexual health and contraceptive choices. It is essential for health professionals to be aware of these influences when supporting a young person in their decision making.

Motivation

There is a general assumption that teenage pregnancy is accidental. It appears to be a young person's failure to understand the risk, inability to obtain contraception or inability to negotiate contraceptive use with their partner that leads to pregnancy. Yet this makes the assumption that all young people are motivated to prevent pregnancy. In fact, some young people may consciously want to become pregnant or simply may not mind being pregnant. They may see pregnancy as a means of achieving adulthood, finding a purpose in life, having someone to love and strengthening their relationship with their sexual partner.[12]

When young people perceive that they have few career or employment prospects, lost opportunities through having a child are not a consideration. Consequently, they are more likely to engage in unprotected sex or be less committed to avoiding pregnancy.[13]

Family and friends

Friends are more likely to be consulted by young people at the beginning of a pregnancy; family members are more important in finalising their decision.[14] Family members and friends can directly influence a young person's choices regarding child bearing. They may actively encourage child bearing or abortion when a young person is faced with the choice of whether to maintain a pregnancy.

Young people will have also observed the choices made around them regarding child bearing and their consequences; this will in turn influence their own choices.

Partner

A young woman's partner can influence whether she becomes pregnant and her decisions once pregnant; they can encourage her to keep the baby as an expression of their love, or put pressure on to have an abortion. For professionals working with young people, it is important to recognise that a young woman's partner is often directly involved in the decision and his influence should be considered when her choices are being discussed.

The couple will not necessarily be in a long-term committed relationship. One study has shown that only half of teenage mothers are still in a relationship with the father a year after the baby's birth; the other half have no steady partner.[15] Hence these men are often distanced from the consequences of teenage pregnancy and are less likely to feel responsible for preventing pregnancy in the future.

Role of professionals working with young people

What is different about countries that have low teen pregnancy rates? They have similar social class variations, education levels and areas of poverty as the UK. However, the differences appear to lie in the following areas:[1]

- an open and accepting attitude to teenage sexuality
- widely available sexual health information and education
- easy access to confidential contraceptive services.

For the professional working with young people, a holistic approach to their sexual health is required. This includes access to accurate and up-to-date information on contraception, abortion and pregnancy and a knowledge of local services providing for young people's sexual health and contraception, pregnancy and counselling. An accepting attitude to young people's sexuality, being willing to talk about sex, raising a young person's self-esteem, and encouraging their ambition and life goals are all vital requirements.

Access to services

Young people want easy access to contraceptive services with hours that suit them, and reassurance that confidentiality will be respected.[16] Hence the timing, environment and staff of young people's clinics are important issues for this client group. Creativity in where services are provided may increase young people's opportunity to access clinics: school nurses are ideally placed to offer sexual health and contraceptive advice in drop-in clinics in schools; sexual health advisers could be present and contraception provided in other clinics such as accident and emergency (A&E); and clinics could be set up in non-clinical environments such as shopping centres and sports complexes. Box 4.3 contains a description of an innovative partnership between a school health service and a youth club.[17]

Box 4.3   Setting up a sexual health clinic in a secondary school[17]

A sexual health service has been set up in a youth club on the site of a school in Trent. The idea originated from teenagers asking their school nurse for condoms after sex education lessons. It is run by the school and a local youth service. A male youth worker runs group work sessions every week; these sessions focus on feelings and relationships and have been particularly popular with young men. School nurses dispense free condoms, emergency contraception and carry out pregnancy testing under protocol.

   With a male youth worker present young men feel more comfortable accessing the service. If young women do not feel comfortable talking to a male worker, the school nurse (who is female) is available.

Sex education

It would be beneficial if all young people delayed sexual activity. This would reduce teenage pregnancy and the prevalence of STIs as well as any negative psychological impact of early sexual relationships. However, it is not enough to simply tell young people not to have sex. In a society where they are constantly surrounded by sexual images, an abstinence message can be confusing and counter-productive. It can result in the perpetuation of myths and mis-information about sex and contraception amongst young people, leading to an increase in unintentional risk-taking behaviour. Young people find themselves in a relationship and do not have the knowledge or skills to negotiate boundaries and prevent STIs and pregnancy. In fact, it has been found that if young people have clear and accurate information regarding sex and contraception before they begin to explore their sexuality, they delay sexual activity. In addition, young people are more likely to practise safe sex when they do become sexually active.[1]

   Similarly, a focus on contraception alone can have detrimental effects. By making contraception more easily available, without a programme of sex education that includes the consequences of early sexual intercourse and the value of intimate relationships, the cost of sexual intercourse to young people is reduced in their eyes. As a consequence their sexual activity can increase. (There is a more detailed description of the research that has revealed these consequences in Chapter 6.) A project in the Lothians that advocates free condoms and emergency contraception to school pupils appears to have led to an increase in pregnancy rates. It has emerged that girls aged between 13 and 15 years in this area are 14% more likely to become pregnant than elsewhere in Scotland. Before the scheme was introduced the figure was 3%.[18] In its defence, it is a long-term project that aims to change attitudes and behaviours, and this can take years to come to fruition.

   Sex education that includes discussion of the emotional aspects of relationships with role playing is helpful in strengthening assertiveness over relationship issues, abstention and contraceptive use (*see* Box 4.4). Negotiation skills for relationships should be incorporated into any work on sexual health with young people. Negotiation skills are an important part of the sex and relationships education (SRE) curriculum, and are useful in all areas of life. (*See* Chapter 10 for more on outreach.)

Box 4.4   Sexual Health Workshops[19]

In Hackney, East London, a group of professionals with a specialist interest in sex education for young people form the SRE team. The team carry out workshops in secondary schools as part of the curriculum.

The workshops focus on contraception, pregnancy, sexual health negotiation skills and sexuality. The workshop entitled 'Choices and Decisions' looks at negotiation skills in the context of the following questions:

- What are we looking for in a relationship?
- When is the right time to have sex?
- How do we talk to the person we are with about sex?
- How do we make positive decisions about who we have sex with?
- What do we do if we fancy someone?
- How do we know if someone fancies us?
- How should we act?
- What is appropriate?
- What should we do if we feel uncomfortable with, or don't like, what is happening?
- How do our cultural beliefs and values affect our choices and decisions in relationships?
- What is sexuality?
- Who are we attracted to and why?
- How do we talk about and feel comfortable with our sexuality?
- How do we get the best out of relationships and where can we get more information?

Active learning methods are used in the workshops and include:

- brainstorming
- scenarios/role play
- yes/no continuum
- drama
- visual aids: pictures/flip charts/video.

The workshops receive a positive response both from teaching staff and pupils. Teaching staff are supported in SRE and the young people feel more confident about choices within sexual relationships, gain new information and enjoy the workshops.

For young women who consciously want to become pregnant, or don't mind getting pregnant, traditional pregnancy prevention programmes may not be effective. Supporting young people in delaying sexual activity, obtaining contraception and negotiating contraceptive use more assertively may not persuade them to avoid putting themselves at risk of pregnancy. Prevention may be more effective if unrealistic positive illusions of teenage child bearing are addressed. This could be done through inviting young parents to talk with teens about their experiences of parenthood or through the increasingly popular 'baby think it over' dolls that simulate what it would be like to have a baby.

'Baby think it over' dolls

'Baby think it over' dolls are a virtual infant simulator designed to give teenagers a realistic experience of caring for a baby. The dolls are scale replicas of three-month-old babies, they weigh 7.5 lb, are anatomically correct and come in different ethnic models. They mimic the unpredictable and often intrusive behaviour of a baby. They require a carer to respond to the baby's cry by simulating feeding, nappy changing and winding 24 hours a day. A computer chip inside the simulator records response times, episodes of neglect and incorrect handling and measures the responses of the carer. The simulator responds to rough or incorrect handling by crying.

The majority of programmes that use the dolls focus on teaching parenting skills and demonstrating the unpredictable, life-changing and time-consuming nature of babies. Many use them in the context of their local teenage pregnancy strategy, in the hope that they will encourage young people to take greater steps to delay pregnancy and parenthood.

Anecdotal evidence suggests that those using the simulator feel they illustrate the strain having a baby would put on their family life, relationships and social life. The majority of young people appear relieved to hand back the baby and determined to postpone child bearing. A small-scale study in a West Midlands school showed that after use of the dolls 31% of students were less positive about their ability to care for a baby and 48% said that they had changed their mind about parenting. Use of the dolls may raise a number of issues; it is recommended that young people should have the opportunity for a one-to-one debrief after taking the simulators home.[20]

Summary

Teenage pregnancy has been identified by the Government as a problem area and it has set targets to reduce levels and the resultant poverty and social exclusion. Although we do compare poorly with other Western countries, teenage pregnancy statistics are improving due to increased knowledge about sexual health and contraception as well as increased availability of abortion.

There are many issues surrounding a young woman's choices regarding pregnancy, including the motivation to avoid pregnancy and the influence of family, friends and partner. The professional working with young people should have an open attitude to young people's sexual health and contraceptive choices. A young person's access to sexual health and contraceptive services should be improved through using innovative locations as well as attention to timing, environment and staff who should be young people-friendly (*see* Chapter 2 for more information on engaging young people). Prevention work should start early; sexual health information should include biological facts as well as work around relationships, self-esteem, negotiation skills and perceived consequences of pregnancy. Prevention work is not restricted to the school curriculum – both professionals and parents can be involved in sexual health promotion with young people (*see* Chapter 10).

References

1   Brook (2003) *Teenage conceptions: statistics and trends.* www.brook.org.uk/content/fact2_TeenageConceptions.pdf
2   Teenage Pregnancy Unit (2004) *Statistics: Conception Statistics for England 1998–2001.* Teenage Pregnancy Unit, London. www.dfes.gov.uk/teenage pregnancy/dsp_content.cfm?pageld = 229
3   www.baby-parenting.co.uk/pregnancy/teen_pregnancy_statistics.html
4   Bull S and Hogu CJR (1998) Exploratory analysis of factors associated with teens repeating child bearing. *Journal of Health Care for the Poor and Underserved.* **9** (1): 42–61.
5   www.doh.gov.uk national statistics, health survey for England. Table 33 – social class of head of household by ethnic group.
6   www.socialexclusionunit.gov.uk
7   www.socialexclusionunit.gov.uk/1999/teenpreg%20summary.htm
8   www.likeitis.org.uk
9   Kiernan K (1995) *Transition to Parenthood: young mothers, young fathers – associated factors and later life experiences.* Welfare State programme. Discussion paper WSP/113. LSE/Suntory and Toyota International Centres for Economics and Related Disciplines, London.
10 Coard SI, Nitz K and Felice ME (2000) Repeat pregnancy among urban adolescents: socio-demographic, family and health factors. *Adolescence.* **35** (137): 193–200.
11 Fu H, Darrock JE, Haas T *et al.* (1999) Contraceptive failure rates: new estimates from the 1995 National Survey of Family Growth. *Family Planning Perspectives.* **31** (2): 56–63.
12 Ford K, Weglicki L, Kershaw T *et al.* (2002) Effects of a prenatal care intervention for adolescent mothers on birth weight, repeat pregnancy and education outcomes at one year postpartum. *Journal of Perinatal Education.* **11** (1): 35–8.
13 Kirby D, Coyle K, Jeffrey B *et al.* (2001) Manifestations of poverty and birth rates among young teenagers in California zip code areas. *Family Planning Perspectives.* **33** (2): 63–9.
14 Evans A (2001) The influence of significant others on Australian teenagers' decisions about pregnancy resolution. *Family Planning Perspectives.* **33** (5): 224–30.
15 Quinlivan JA, Petersen RW and Gurrin LC (1999) Adolescent pregnancy: psychopathology missed. *Australian and New Zealand Journal of Psychiatry.* **33**: 864–8.
16 Bekaert S (2003) Developing adolescent services in general practice. *Nursing Standard.* **17** (36): 33–6.
17 www.innovate.org.uk/hvsn/
18 Editorial (2004) Approach to tackling teenage pregnancy branded a costly flop. *The Herald,* 12 April.
19 Bekaert S (2002) Sexual health workshops. *Paediatric Nursing.* **14** (4): 22–5.
20 Pickles J (2000) 'Baby think it over' electronic simulators: are they effective? *Journal of School Health.* **71** (5): 188–95.

Resources
For young people

* *Marie Stopes International* and the *British Pregnancy Advisory Service* are private organisations that provide information about abortion, contraception and sexual health. They also take termination referrals. They can be contacted online or by telephone:
www.mariestopes.org.uk; Tel: 0845 300 1212
www.bpas.org; Tel: 08457 30 40 30

* *Abortion: just so you know*
Leaflet providing information on abortion aimed at young people.
Available from the Family Planning Association (fpa) direct: PO Box 1078, East Oxford DO, Oxford OX4 6JE. Tel: 01865 719418. www.fpa.org.uk/about/pubs

For professionals

* www.teenagepregnancyunit.gov.uk
The Teenage Pregnancy Unit is a cross-Government unit, located within the Department for Education and Skills, which was set up to implement the Social Exclusion Unit's report on teenage pregnancy. This website contains information about the Government's Teenage Pregnancy Strategy, including guidance issued by the Teenage Pregnancy Unit as well as relevant publications from other Government departments. There is also information about local implementation of the strategy and details about the Independent Advisory Group on Teenage Pregnancy.

* www.brook.org.uk
Brook runs a unique network of 17 centres across the UK, providing contraception, advice and sexual health counselling to young people as well as outreach, education and satellite services in response to local need.
    It also runs a national Young People's Information Service which informs young people about sexual health services in their area. This provides basic information and support on sexual health topics such as contraception, emergency contraception, pregnancy testing, abortion and STIs. People can ring the freephone helpline (0800 0185 023) or send a question through 'Ask Brook', a confidential online enquiry service, via the Brook website. They can also get details of local services texted direct to their mobile phone.
    Brook also produces a range of publications for use by teachers, parents, youth workers and young people themselves on a variety of sexual health issues. Its website contains information regarding sexual health and pregnancy for both professionals and young people.

* www.btio.com
American site dedicated to information about 'baby think it over' dolls.

* www.lifechoice.co.uk
The official UK distributor and supplier of 'baby think it over' dolls.

CHAPTER 5

Young people and contraception

This chapter provides basic information on the male and female reproductive systems, periods, contraceptive methods and contraceptive myths.

A sexually active young woman who does not use contraception has a 90% chance of conceiving within a year.[1] Yet contraception isn't always high on the agenda when young people become sexually active. Various pregnancy myths such as 'it's ok on my period' or 'not on the first time' persist. Young people worry over confidentiality, knowing where to access contraception and whether it is legal to use contraception. This stops them asking for contraceptive advice. They are afraid of the effect hormonal contraception may have on them, they don't always understand how to use the method, and their partner doesn't always support them in seeking or using contraception. Young people are generally poor contraception users and delay seeking advice until crisis management is required. Even when they use a contraceptive method, the failure rates are higher than for older women.

A study of 14–19 year-olds who had had an abortion or a previous negative pregnancy test showed that 75% of both groups selected reliable contraception after their visit to a contraception clinic. However, only 10.3% and 5.8% respectively were using reliable contraception at a subsequent appointment.

The implant and injectables have the lowest failure rates (2–3%), followed by the pill (8%), the diaphragm and cervical cap (12%), the male condom (14%), periodic abstinence (21%), withdrawal (24%) and spermicides (26%).[2]

According to these failure rates, implants and injections are the most effective methods of contraception for young people. This is probably because they do not rely on the user having to remember to take tablets or use protection when having sex. The intrauterine device (IUD) was not included in this research because although it can be fitted after an abortion, it would not be routinely suggested after a pregnancy test.

The IUD is not routinely offered to young women as a contraceptive method for several reasons:

- it is more difficult to fit an IUD in a woman who has not had a vaginal delivery
- it is an invasive procedure

- the pregnancy test may not be conclusive and an IUD fitted in a pregnant woman may disrupt the pregnancy
- it is preferred for a woman with a regular partner and low risk of contracting a sexually transmitted infection (STI), as some STIs can track up the threads of the IUD and cause pelvic inflammatory disease (PID).

A recent addition to the range of contraceptive methods is the hormone patch. It may prove to be a good contraceptive method for young people as it is non-invasive and only requires the user to change the patch three times a month. This may be easier than the method it most closely resembles, the combined pill, where the user has to remember to take a tablet every day for 21 days.

Role of the health professional

Health professionals working with young people but who are not contraception practitioners must have an accurate and up-to-date basic knowledge of contraceptive methods and be able to dispel myths surrounding contraception and pregnancy. It is important to know where to direct young people when they need expert advice and/or access to contraceptive services.

Male reproductive organs

The main function of the male reproductive organs (*see* Figure 5.1) is to make sperm and pass them to the female. The system consists of two round glands

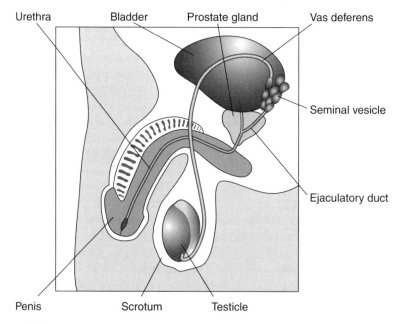

Figure 5.1 Male reproductive organs.

called testicles, or testes, that lie in a special sac (scrotum) outside the body. Within the testes are tubules and ducts where sperm are produced. A duct, called the vas deferens, comes out of each testicle and up into the pelvis. At this point the seminal vesicle joins the vas deferens. The seminal vesicle adds seminal fluid to the sperm. The duct then becomes the ejaculatory duct that fuses with the urethra (which carries urine) at the prostate gland. The duct is then called the prostatic urethra and carries both urine and semen through the penis. The penis is made up of vascular spaces and erectile tissue.

Female reproductive system

The female reproductive system (*see* Figure 5.2) is designed to make eggs, favour fertilisation and nurture the growing fetus during pregnancy. The ovaries produce

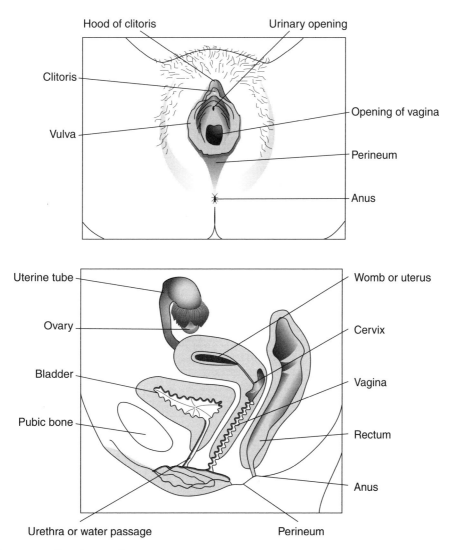

Figure 5.2   Female reproductive system.

eggs (or ova) from follicles. The egg travels down the uterine tubes to the uterus where, if fertilised, it can implant and the fetus develop (see below). At the base of the uterus is the cervix leading to the vagina where sperm can be introduced from the penis.

Fertilisation

Fertilisation takes place when a sperm and egg fuse. Once a month an egg is released from the ovaries (ovulation) and travels down the uterine tubes. If it meets sperm in the uterine tubes it may be fertilised. The fertilised egg then travels to the uterus and implants in the uterine wall where the fetus develops.

Ectopic pregnancy

Ectopic pregnancy is where a fetus develops outside the uterus, most commonly in the uterine tube. This occurs when the passage of a fertilised egg down the tube is impaired, e.g. through PID that has left scar tissue on the tubes. The signs of an ectopic pregnancy are one or two missed periods, bleeding and acute abdominal pain. Unless it is removed it can rupture the tube and can be fatal.

Ectopic pregnancy is an acute condition that usually results in hospital treatment. In England it accounts for 10% of the deaths that result from complications of pregnancy and childbirth. Chlamydia causes 43% of ectopic pregnancies. It is a sexually transmitted infection that, if left untreated, can damage the uterine tubes (*see* Chapter 7 for more details on chlamydia). This impedes the passage of eggs (ova) down the tubes and if a fertilised egg implants in the uterine tube rather than the uterus an ectopic pregnancy results.

The incidence of ectopic pregnancy has risen since the mid 1980s. This may be because an increasing number of women are becoming pregnant later in life, when the risk of ectopic pregnancy is higher due to the cumulative risk over time of damage to the upper reproductive tract from STIs and PID. In 1997, the incidence of ectopic pregnancy in women aged 40 years or over was seven times that in women aged 17–19 years. (Between 1990 and 1997, the number of births to women aged 35–39 and 30–34 rose by 44% and 20% respectively; and fell by 20%, 34% and 17% in the 25–29, 20–24 and under 20 age groups respectively.)[3]

Periods

Before contraception can be understood it is helpful to have an understanding of the menstrual cycle as most hormonal contraceptive methods interrupt this cycle in some way.

The menstrual cycle is from the first day of a period until the day before the next period starts (*see* Figure 5.3). Its length varies for each individual and often from one period to the next. It can be as short as 21 days and as long as 40 days.

The menstrual cycle is controlled by hormones. The chemical messenger follicle-stimulating hormone-releasing factor (FSH-RF) is released by the hypothalamus, a

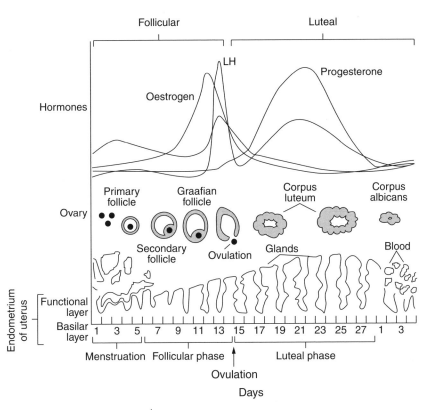

Figure 5.3   The menstrual cycle.[4]

gland in the brain. This hormone tells the pituitary, also in the brain, to secrete follicle stimulating hormone (FSH) and luteinising hormone (LH) into the bloodstream. These hormones cause the follicles in the ovaries to begin to mature.

The maturing follicles release the hormone oestrogen. Oestrogen causes the lining of the uterus to thicken. When the oestrogen level reaches a certain point it causes the hypothalamus to release luteinising hormone-releasing factor (LH-RF), causing the pituitary to release a large amount of LH. This surge of LH triggers the most mature follicle to burst open and release an egg. This is called ovulation. (Many birth-control pills work by blocking this LH surge and inhibiting the release of an egg.)

Inside the uterine tube, the egg is carried towards the uterus. Fertilisation may occur if sperm are present as the egg reaches the uterus.

The follicle from which the egg burst becomes the corpus luteum (yellow body). As it heals, it produces the hormones oestrogen and, in larger amounts, progesterone, which is necessary for the maintenance of a pregnancy. Progesterone causes the surface of the uterine lining (the endometrium) to become covered with mucus, secreted from glands within the lining itself. If fertilisation and implantation do not occur, levels of progesterone drop, causing the arteries of the lining to close off, stopping blood flow to the surface of the lining. The lining of endometrium comes away as a period.

The drop in hormones from the ovaries stimulates the hypothalamus and pituitary gland to begin to release FSH and start the next cycle.

Forms of contraception

Hormonal and intrauterine contraception is available through dedicated community contraception and sexual health clinics, departments of sexual health within hospitals (sometimes called genito-urinary medicine services – GUM) and general practice surgeries. Emergency contraception only is available through additional sources such as A&E departments, some school nurses and over the counter at pharmacies. Condoms are available from contraception and sexual health clinics, various commercial outlets (usually pharmacies), some bars and nightclubs, some GPs and various community schemes.

The following are concise descriptions of contraceptive methods – their advantages, disadvantages, side effects and contraindications. If a fuller description is desired by the reader, please refer to one of the recommended texts in the resources section.

Male condom

Efficacy
The male condom is 98% effective.

How does it work?
It is put over an erect penis to catch sperm and prevent them entering the vagina.

Advantages
As well as stopping pregnancy, condoms (including Femidom) are the only method that also protects against STIs.

Condoms come in many different varieties. They can be different flavours and colours, ribbed or smooth, come with or without spermicide, be made of latex or polyurethane and range from sensitive to extra strong.

Disadvantages
- Condom use must be negotiated between both partners.
- May be seen as interrupting sex.

Contraindications
Allergy to latex or spermicide.

Possible problems
- Burst, split or slipped condom during sexual intercourse.
- Allergy to the condom.
- Loss of sensation.

How to use a condom[5]

| Step 1 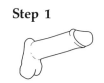 | Check for (CE)* mark – the European standard mark (indication of quality standard; has been tested).

Check the condom is in date. |

Check for tears and rips in the packet. Any hole in the packet will mean the condom has dried out and may split. It is best to keep condoms in a dry, cool place.

Put the condom on when the penis is erect, before there is any contact between the penis and your partner's body. Fluid released from the penis during the early stages of an erection (pre-ejaculate) can contain sperm.

Step 2

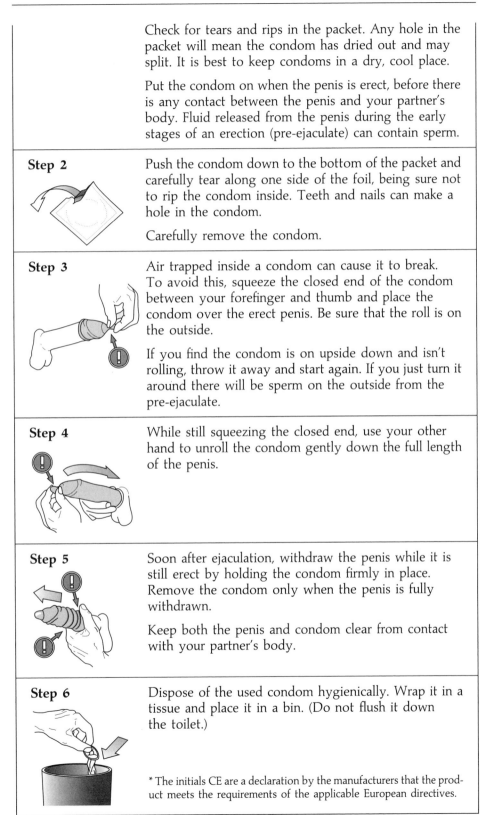

Push the condom down to the bottom of the packet and carefully tear along one side of the foil, being sure not to rip the condom inside. Teeth and nails can make a hole in the condom.

Carefully remove the condom.

Step 3

Air trapped inside a condom can cause it to break. To avoid this, squeeze the closed end of the condom between your forefinger and thumb and place the condom over the erect penis. Be sure that the roll is on the outside.

If you find the condom is on upside down and isn't rolling, throw it away and start again. If you just turn it around there will be sperm on the outside from the pre-ejaculate.

Step 4

While still squeezing the closed end, use your other hand to unroll the condom gently down the full length of the penis.

Step 5

Soon after ejaculation, withdraw the penis while it is still erect by holding the condom firmly in place. Remove the condom only when the penis is fully withdrawn.

Keep both the penis and condom clear from contact with your partner's body.

Step 6

Dispose of the used condom hygienically. Wrap it in a tissue and place it in a bin. (Do not flush it down the toilet.)

* The initials CE are a declaration by the manufacturers that the product meets the requirements of the applicable European directives.

Female condom: Femidom®

Efficacy
The female condom is 95% effective.

How does it work?
Femidom is a pre-lubricated, soft, polyurethane sheath that lines the vagina and acts as a barrier to sperm entering the vagina. There is a smaller inner ring and larger outer ring. The smaller inner ring is used to feed the Femidom into the vagina. Most of the Femidom goes inside the woman and the larger ring overlaps the outer area of the vagina.

Advantages
• The woman has control over its use.
• It protects against STIs.

Disadvantages
• Some people find them noisy.
• May be seen as interrupting sex.

Contraindications
Allergy to spermicide.

Possible problems
• The penis may be mistakenly inserted outside the female condom.
• Noise – some women have commented about a rustling noise.

How to use a Femidom[6]

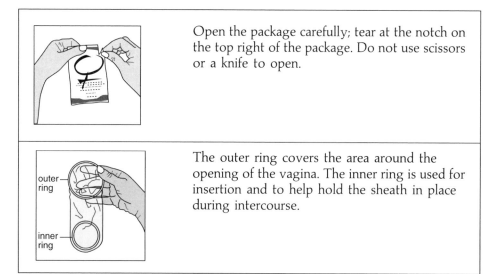

	Open the package carefully; tear at the notch on the top right of the package. Do not use scissors or a knife to open.
outer ring / inner ring	The outer ring covers the area around the opening of the vagina. The inner ring is used for insertion and to help hold the sheath in place during intercourse.

While holding the sheath at the closed end, grasp the flexible inner ring and squeeze it with the thumb and second or middle finger so it becomes long and narrow.

Choose a position that is comfortable for insertion — squat, raise one leg, sit or lie down.

Gently insert the inner ring into the vagina. Feel the inner ring go up and move into place.

Place the index finger on the inside of the condom and push the inner ring up as far as it will go. Be sure the sheath is not twisted. The outer ring should remain on the outside of the vagina.

The female condom is now in place and ready for use with your partner.

When you are ready, gently guide your partner's penis into the sheath's opening with your hand to make sure that it enters properly — be sure that the penis is not entering on the side, between the sheath and the vaginal wall.

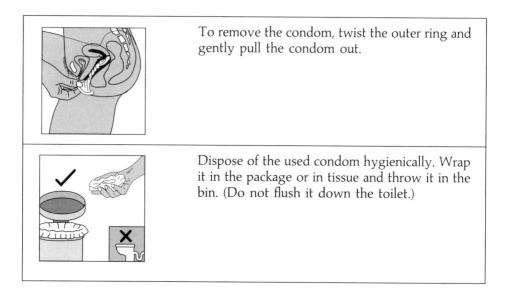

| | To remove the condom, twist the outer ring and gently pull the condom out. |
| | Dispose of the used condom hygienically. Wrap it in the package or in tissue and throw it in the bin. (Do not flush it down the toilet.) |

Ideally, the 'Double Dutch' method should be recommended. This is where the young woman uses a reliable form of hormonal contraception as well as condoms, just in case the condom splits or comes off.

Spermicide

Efficacy
Poor when used alone.

How does it work?
This is a foam, cream or jelly that kills sperm. It is not very effective at preventing pregnancy when used on its own. It is usually used as a lubricant and back-up to the main barrier method, i.e. diaphragm or condom.

Advantages
• Lubricates.
• Easily available.
• Can be used with barrier methods of contraception.

Disadvantages
• Some find it messy.
• Not highly effective when used alone.

Contraindications
Allergy to spermicide.

Side effects
Local irritation.

The combined oral contraceptive pill

Efficacy
The combined pill is over 99% effective if taken according to instructions.

How does it work?
The combined pill contains hormones that copy our natural hormones (oestrogen and progesterone). The combined pill stops ovulation and makes cervical mucus thicker, which stops sperm reaching an egg. Pills are taken for three weeks, followed by a week's break. During the break there is usually a short, light bleed. This is not an actual period but what is called a withdrawal bleed, caused by the level of hormones dropping while the pill is not being taken.

This pill should be taken at the same time every day, but if forgotten it can be taken up to 12 hours later. If more than 12 hours elapse, it should be taken as soon as remembered and condoms used for the following seven days as well as carrying on with the pills. Research has shown that after nine days of not taking the combined pill the ovaries can release an egg. If more than one pill is missed throughout a packet, attendance at a clinic is recommended to check out whether there is any possibility an egg may have been released and whether emergency contraception is required.

Some medication can stop the pill working. Most commonly, antibiotics may interfere with its efficacy. The pill should be continued, but condoms should also be used until seven days after the antibiotics have finished. Diarrhoea and vomiting interfere with absorption in the gut and can stop the pill working; again, condoms should be used during the illness and for seven days after.

Advantages
- The user is in control of the method.
- There is a quick return of fertility after ceasing to use.
- It often makes bleeds lighter and less painful.
- The combined pill is protective against womb and ovarian cancer.

Disadvantages
- The user is in control of the method – it needs to be taken regularly to be effective.
- Rare side effects may include blood clots and increased incidence of breast cancer and cervical cancer.

Contraindications
- Pregnancy
- Breast feeding
- Undiagnosed vaginal or uterine bleeding
- Past or present venous or arterial thrombosis
- Cardiovascular and ischaemic heart disease
- Lipid disorders
- Focal migraines
- Cerebral haemorrhage

- Active liver disease
- Oestrogen-dependent neoplasms
- Obesity (body mass index [BMI] greater than $35 \, kg/m^2$)
- Severe diabetes mellitus with complications
- Smokers over the age of 35
- Family history of arterial or venous disease in a first-degree relative under 45 years
- Acute episodes of Crohn's disease and ulcerative colitis

Relative contraindications
- Sickle cell disease
- Severe depression
- Inflammatory bowel disease in remission
- Diseases where high-density lipoprotein is reduced, e.g. diabetes
- Splenectomy
- Diseases where drug treatment affects the efficacy of the combined pill, e.g. tuberculosis, epilepsy
- Diabetes mellitus
- Obesity (BMI between 30 and $35 \, kg/m^2$)

Possible side effects
- Nausea
- Breast tenderness and swelling
- Breakthrough bleeding
- Depression
- Changes in libido

The hormone patch

Efficacy
The contraceptive patch is 99% effective.

How does it work?
The patch contains oestrogen and a progestogen. The hormones are absorbed through the skin and stop ovulation. The patch can be put on the arm, thigh, back shoulder or buttock. One patch is worn each week for three weeks followed by a patch-free week.

The patch is very sticky and unlikely to come off. However, if it does, or a patch change is forgotten, advice should be sought at a clinic and condoms used until advised.

The manufacturer advises the following:[7]

- If the patch change day is delayed by less than two days, the patch should be changed and the patch change day remains the same.
- If the patch change day is more than 48 hours late, a new patch should be put on and a new four-week cycle begun, with a new patch change day. Condoms should be used for the next seven days.

- If the third patch in a cycle is left on into the patch-free week, the patch should be removed once remembered and a new cycle started at the normal time.
- If the patch-free interval is extended beyond seven days, similarly to the combined pill it is assumed that an egg may have been released after nine days and emergency contraception is needed.

Advantages
- Some side effects may be less than with the combined pill as the hormones are released straight into the bloodstream rather than having to go through the liver first.
- Only three patch changes per cycle.
- The user is in control of the method.
- There is a quick return of fertility after ceasing to use.
- It often makes bleeds lighter and less painful.
- As it is similar to the combined pill, the patch may be protective against womb and ovarian cancer.
- Daily activities such as bathing, showering, swimming and exercise can all be continued as normal without the patch coming off.

Disadvantages
- The user is in control of the method – it needs to be changed at weekly intervals to be effective.
- As the hormones are similar to the combined pill, rare side effects such as blood clots and cancers are the same.

Contraindications
As for the combined pill.

Possible side effects
As for the combined pill plus application site reactions.

The progestogen-only pill

Efficacy
The progestogen-only pill (POP) is 99% effective if taken according to instructions.

How does it work?
The progestogen thickens cervical mucus to stop sperm reaching an egg. In some women it stops ovulation.

This pill is taken every day without a break. It must be taken at the same time every day and will not work if taken over three hours late. After this time the mucus plug at the cervix comes away. If a pill is forgotten and it is more than three hours late, it should be taken as soon as remembered, but condoms should also be used for the next seven days until a protective level of hormone is reached.

Some drugs may interfere with the efficacy of the POP. If the doctor prescribes you any medication it is always best to check it doesn't interfere with the POP.

Vomiting within three hours of taking the POP may stop it working. Again, use condoms for the following seven days as well as taking the pills.

Advantages
- The user is in control of the method.
- There is a quick return of fertility after ceasing to use.
- It can be used whilst breast feeding.
- It is suitable for women who are unable to use the combined pill.

Disadvantages
- The user is in control of the method – it needs to be taken carefully.
- Periods may be irregular.

Contraindications
- Pregnancy
- Undiagnosed genital tract bleeding
- Past or present severe arterial disease
- Severe lipid abnormalities
- Recent trophoblastic disease
- Previous ectopic pregnancy
- Present liver condition

Possible side effects
- Functional ovarian cysts
- Breast tenderness
- Feeling bloated
- Depression
- Variations in weight
- Nausea
- Irregular/no bleeding

Hormone injection

Efficacy
The Depo-Provera® injection is over 99% effective.

How does it work?
The injection contains one hormone, a progestogen, and stops ovulation. An injection is given, usually in the buttock (although it can be given in the arm or thigh), once every 12 weeks. Some drugs can reduce the efficacy of the injection – if the doctor prescribes you any medication it is always best to check it doesn't interfere with the Depo-Provera injection.

Advantages
- One injection every 12 weeks.
- User not involved.
- This method usually stops periods (it keeps the womb lining at the same thickness so there is no build-up of blood).

Disadvantages
- There may be some irregular bleeding or spotting initially.
- Once given it cannot be withdrawn.

• After stopping the injection it can take up to a year for ovulation to reoccur; however, some women ovulate soon after an injection is due.

Contraindications
• Pregnancy
• Undiagnosed genital tract bleeding
• Past or present severe arterial disease
• Severe lipid abnormalities
• Recent trophoblastic disease
• Present liver condition
• Severe depression

Possible side effects
• Headaches
• Feeling bloated
• Depression
• Weight gain
• Mood swings
• Irregular/no bleeding

Intrauterine device

Efficacy
The intrauterine device (IUD) is 98% to over 99% effective.

How does it work?
The IUD is a small plastic device shaped like a T, with thin copper wire wrapped around it. It sits in the uterus and is fitted by a doctor or nurse. The copper impairs the viability of sperm and eggs by altering the uterine fluids, which stops them meeting. The IUD lasts for up to ten years, although it can be taken out at any time.

It is a commonly held belief that an IUD can't be fitted if a woman has not had children; this is not the case. The IUD *is* a contraceptive choice for women who have not had children. It is also routinely fitted as a form of emergency contraception up to five days after unprotected sex, again often in young women who have not had children. The reasoning behind the IUD not being routinely offered to young women is that the threads of the IUD can act as a channel for infection. This infection may cause PID which can affect fertility in the future. A young person is less likely to be settled with one person and therefore more at risk of catching an STI. It can also be more difficult for an IUD to be fitted as the cervix has not been stretched through childbirth.

Advantages
• Works immediately.
• No hormones involved.
• Immediately reversible.
• User not involved.

Disadvantages
• The threads that come out from your cervix can be a channel for infection to track up to the womb.

- It can make periods heavier and longer.
- It needs to be inserted and removed by a doctor or nurse.

Contraindications
- Pregnancy
- Undiagnosed genital tract bleeding
- Previous ectopic pregnancy
- Pelvic or vaginal infection
- Abnormalities of the uterus
- Allergy to components of IUD
- Wilson's disease
- Heavy painful periods
- Fibroids/endometriosis

Possible side effects
- Heavier, more painful periods
- Increased risk of ectopic pregnancy if IUD fails
- Increased risk of pelvic infection
- Malposition or expulsion of IUD
- Pregnancy due to malposition or expulsion of IUD

Intrauterine system: Mirena®

Efficacy
The intrauterine system (IUS) is over 99% effective.

How does it work?
The IUS is a small plastic device with slow-releasing progestogen in the stem. It sits in the uterus and is inserted and removed by a doctor or nurse. The progestogen hormone used is called levonorgestrel and it works by thickening the cervical mucus to stop sperm reaching an egg. It also makes the womb lining unfavourable to implantation. It works for up to five years. Mirena is not effective as emergency contraception.

Advantages
- Works immediately.
- User not involved.
- Periods will be much lighter, shorter and less painful.
- Periods may stop.

Disadvantages
- There may be some irregular bleeding.
- It needs to be inserted and removed by a specially trained doctor or nurse.

Contraindications
- Pregnancy
- Undiagnosed genital tract bleeding

- Abnormalities of the uterus
- Uterine or cervical malignancy
- Liver condition

Possible side effects
- Breast tenderness
- Acne
- Headaches
- Feeling bloated
- Mood changes
- Nausea
- Irregular/no bleeding

Implant

Efficacy
The implant is over 99% effective.

How does it work?
The implant is a small, soft tube, the size of a matchstick, that is inserted by a doctor or nurse under the skin of the upper arm. It is not visible but can be felt under the skin. Like the injection it releases a small amount of progestogen every day; this stops ovulation and makes cervical mucus thicker, preventing sperm from getting through. It lasts for three years.

Advantages
- Works immediately.
- User not involved.

Disadvantages
- Bleeding pattern can be unpredictable.
- It needs to be inserted and removed by a doctor or nurse.

Contraindications
- Pregnancy
- Undiagnosed vaginal bleeding
- Severe arterial disease
- Liver adenoma

Possible side effects
- Irregular or no bleeding
- Nausea
- Vomiting
- Headache
- Dizziness
- Breast discomfort
- Depression
- Skin disorders
- Disturbance of appetite/weight changes

- Changes in libido
- Alopecia

Diaphragm

Efficacy
The diaphragm is 92% to 96% effective if used according to instructions.

How does it work?
This is a round dome made of rubber that is used with spermicide. It goes inside the vagina and covers the cervix. It is a barrier to sperm getting into the cervix and reaching an egg.

Advantages
- The woman is in control of the method.
- No hormones involved.
- Provides lubrication.

Disadvantages
- Some people find it messy.
- User has to be motivated to use it.
- Need to be able to find own cervix to check diaphragm is in right place.

Contraindications
Allergic reaction to spermicide.

Side effects
Local irritation.

How to use a diaphragm[8]

(a)

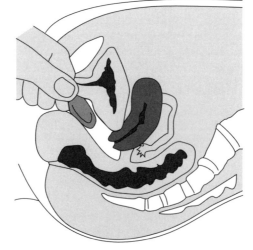

Figure 5.4 (a) Diaphragm being inserted; (b) Checking the position of the diaphragm.[8]

(b)

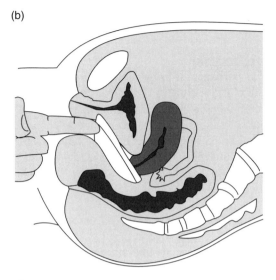

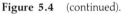

Figure 5.4   (continued).

The emergency pill

Efficacy
The emergency pill can be taken up to three days (72 hours) after unprotected sexual intercourse – it is more effective the sooner it is taken. It is 95% effective if taken within 24 hours after unprotected sex, 85% within 25–48 hours.[9]

How does it work?
The emergency pill contains progestogen. Depending on where in the woman's cycle it is taken, it either delays ovulation so there is no egg for the sperm to reach or, if there is a fertilised egg, stops it implanting.

Advantages
- Effective at preventing pregnancy.
- The woman is in control of the method.
- It can be used after unprotected sexual intercourse.

Disadvantages
- It doesn't provide future contraception.
- May disrupt the next period.
- It is less effective the later it is taken after unprotected sexual intercourse.

Contraindications
- Its effectiveness can be reduced by enzyme-inducing drugs.

Possible side effects
- Nausea and vomiting
- Breast tenderness
- Headache
- Dizziness

- Fatigue
- Bleeding patterns may be temporarily disturbed

A note on the emergency pill

The emergency pill is perhaps the most controversial method of contraception. Some groups have called it the abortion pill, though technically it doesn't cause an abortion as despite there being a fertilised egg, it has not implanted. Many fear that its increased availability will encourage young people to have sex. However, research has shown that increased knowledge of sex and availability of contraception do not encourage young people to have sex earlier, in fact it has the opposite effect (*see* Chapter 10 for further details). In addition, it is debatable whether the emergency pill has become more available to young people as it costs over £20 from a chemist, and pharmacists cannot supply it to under-16s. School nurses are ideally placed to provide emergency contraception, but they are not all able to do so (see below).

However, young people are accessing emergency contraception from clinics and general practice surgeries. Figures suggest that teenagers' use of emergency contraception has increased in recent years. The number of occasions when emergency contraception was provided to girls under 16 in family planning clinics in England increased from 3000 in 1990–91 to nearly 20 000 in 1996–97, and from 15 000 to 66 700 for women aged 16–19.[1]

Issuing hormonal contraception via Patient Group Directions

Nurses and pharmacists are able to dispense hormonal methods of contraception as long as they have received training and are signed up to a 'Patient Group Direction'.

Patient Group Directions (PGDs) are documents that make it legal for medicines to be given to groups of patients without individual prescriptions. Professionals signed up to the PGD can give the medicine as long as the client fits the PGD criteria, otherwise they need to be referred to a doctor. This has increased the availability of hormonal emergency contraception.

PGDs have enabled nurses to dispense most methods of contraception within contraception clinics and general practice surgeries; and some school nurses and pharmacists have been issuing the emergency contraception pill via PGDs.

School nurses providing emergency contraception in schools was an idea floated by the Teenage Pregnancy Strategy. The accessibility of school nurses to young people together with their training and duty of confidentiality mean they are an ideal professional body to provide contraceptive advice and emergency contraception. It has been difficult for all school nurses to fulfil this role due to lack of training in this area, workload and opposition from some parents, teachers and governors, but some have successfully set up such a service. A drop-in service in a senior school in south Derbyshire is one such example (*see* Box 5.1).

Box 5.1   Issuing emergency contraception in a senior school in south Derbyshire

Making emergency contraception available in a senior school in South Derbyshire is part of a pilot project in the county to develop outreach sexual health clinics for young people requiring emergency contraception following unprotected sexual intercourse, but who cannot easily access town centre sites. The school has a wide and largely rural catchment area with some of the villages having limited access to public services. This initiative was intended to enhance an existing 'drop-in' service in school where the school nurse was available to provide advice and counselling on a range of topics, including physical, psychological and mental health as well as a variety of social issues.

Following consultation with the headteacher and governing body, a unanimous decision was reached that the school nurse would be able to issue emergency contraception, thus enhancing an already comprehensive sex and relationships educational programme.

After discussion with the governing body, parents were consulted and advised of the proposal. It was stressed that the school nurse, while offering a confidential service to underage sexually active students, would strongly encourage discussion with their parents. Child protection issues and Fraser Guidelines competence would remain paramount. Issues around peer pressure and the right to say 'no' would be discussed and the students would be offered follow-up appointments.

The school nurse is able to issue emergency contraception under a Patient Group Direction approved by the primary care trust and always has access to a family planning clinic. A comprehensive personal and familial medical history is taken as well as the reason for obtaining emergency contraception.

To date, a number of students have requested emergency contraception. They have said they appreciate the service because of its user-friendliness and accessibility. An unexpected outcome has been the number of students requesting advice about sexually transmitted infections.[10]

Over-the-counter emergency contraception

Recently, the emergency contraceptive pill has been available for women aged 16 and above to buy from pharmacists without prescription. Although the elevated price excludes younger people or poorer women with little spare cash, the added route by which women can obtain hormonal emergency contraception is welcome.

There is no protocol for pharmacists supplying the emergency contraceptive pill, but recommendations for the best practice have been set out by the Royal Pharmaceutical Society. These include the following:[11]

- Pharmacists should deal with the request personally and decide whether to supply the product or refer the client to an appropriate healthcare professional.
- Pharmacists should ensure that all necessary advice and information are provided to enable the client to assess whether to use the product.
- Requests for emergency hormonal contraception should be handled sensitively with due regard being given to the customer's right to privacy.
- Pharmacists should whenever possible take reasonable measures to inform patients of regular methods of contraception, disease prevention and sources of help.

Consideration needs to be given to training, time constraints and whether privacy is available in the pharmacy.

Common myths about contraception

There are all sorts of weird and wonderful contraception myths that are popular amongst young people: putting a watch around your penis before sex means the radioactivity of the dial kills off sperm; a Coca-Cola vaginal douche; standing on a telephone directory and drinking a lot of milk all stop pregnancy. Other myths include thinking you can't get pregnant if you stay upside down for two hours after sex; cough immediately after sex; or have sex in the bath, on a boat or with your clothes on. The myths that come up frequently during consultations with young people are dealt with here in more detail.

'You can't get pregnant if you are on your period.' It is possible to become pregnant whilst on your period. A woman releases an egg approximately 14 days before her period. If there are 28 days from one period to another, this will mean she releases an egg on day 14 of her cycle (day one being the first day of her period). Sperm can live up to seven days and the egg for three, so there are ten days when a woman could become pregnant. If a woman's period is more than seven days long with a 28-day cycle, she may well be still bleeding on one of the risky days. If a woman has a shorter cycle than 28 days, she could become pregnant whilst on her period.

   However, this formula should not be relied upon. Many things can affect the timing of ovulation; even if a woman has a very regular cycle the formula above may not always be accurate. It is always better to use a reliable method of contraception if pregnancy is to be avoided.

'We use the withdrawal method.' From the moment of arousal the man produces pre-ejaculate. This is mainly for lubrication, to make it easier for the penis to go inside the woman. But it has thousands of sperm in it as well; so even though the man withdraws before ejaculation there is already a lot of sperm inside the vagina that could reach and fertilise an egg.

'You can't get pregnant the first time.' Regardless of whether it is the first time, sperm can fertilise an egg.

'The pill/injection/coil will stop me from having children when I am older.' All methods of hormonal contraception are reversible. There are no long-term effects on a woman's fertility if she has used a hormonal method of contraception. The IUD stops working as soon as it is removed.

'The pill makes you put on weight.' Recent studies have shown that this is not the case and any weight gain that you observe when someone is taking the pill for months to years is a natural weight gain.[12]

'It is harmful to take the emergency pill too many times.' It is safe to take the emergency pill as many times as needed; there will be no negative effects on your body or fertility. What it can do, however, is interrupt your periods, so if it is taken many times close together it is very difficult to know when ovulation might occur and unprotected sex is therefore very risky. In addition, the emergency contraceptive pill is not 100% effective and it would be better to use a reliable ongoing method of contraception to avoid the uncertainty and inconvenience of using the emergency pill many times.

Summary

All too often teenagers seek contraceptive advice at the crisis management stage. It is the role of the health professional to have accurate and up-to-date knowledge of contraceptive methods and myths surrounding conception and contraception to be able to promote safe sex and contraception use. It is important to know where young people can access local contraceptive services. The resources listed at the end of the chapter can support a health promotion session on contraception or be made available for young people to access informally, e.g. in toilets, a leaflet rack, etc.

References

1   Brook Advisory (2003) *Teenage Conceptions: statistics and trends.* www.brook. org.uk/content/fact2_TeenageConceptions.pdf

2   Fu H, Darroch J, Haas T *et al.* (1999) Contraceptive failure rates: new estimates from the 1995 National Survey of Family Growth. *Family Planning Perspectives.* **31** (2): 56–63.

3   Health Development Agency (2000) Sexually transmitted diseases quarterly report: genital chlamydia infection, ectopic pregnancy and syphilis in England and Wales. *Communicable Diseases Report.* **10** (13): 116.

4   Everett S (2000) *Handbook of Contraception and Family Planning*, p. 15. Ballière-Tindall, Edinburgh.

5   www.feelconfident.co.uk/condoms/how_to_put_on_a_condom.htm

6   www.eros.shop.co.uk/how_to_use_a_femidom_guide.html

7   www.janssen-cilag.co.uk/product/pdf/pil100121.pdf

8   Everett S (2000) *Handbook of Contraception and Family Planning*, pp. 66–7. Ballière-Tindall, Edinburgh.

9   www.mariestopes.org.uk/ww/contraception-emergency.htm

10 Department of Health. *Innovate NHS.* www.innovate.had-online.org.uk

11 Practice guidance on the supply of emergency hormonal contraception as a pharmacy medicine: www.rpsgb.org.uk/pdfs.ehcguid.pdf

12 Wilkinson C and Szarewski A (2003) *Contraceptive Dilemmas.* Altman, St Albans.

Resources
For young people

- *4 Girls: a below-the-bra guide to the female body*
  A Family Planning Association (fpa) A6 booklet which covers: sexual development; feelings; weight; diet; body hair; breasts; genitals; menstrual cycle; sexual health; contraception; STIs; what to do if you think you might be pregnant.

- *4 Boys: a below-the-belt guide to the male body*
  An fpa A6 booklet which covers: body changes; the male reproductive system; self-examination; masturbation; ejaculation; condoms.

- *Periods: what you need to know*
  An fpa A6 booklet which covers: reproductive system; periods; frequently asked questions re periods; sanitary towels and tampons; activities when on period.

- *Is everybody doing it? Your guide to contraception*
  An fpa A6 booklet which covers: are you ready to have sex? Where to get information and help about contraception; brief information on STIs; condom use; contraceptive methods; what to do if you think you might be pregnant.

All the above titles are available from the fpa direct: PO Box 1078, East Oxford DO, Oxford OX4 6JE. Tel: 01865 719418. www.fpa.org.uk/about/pubs

- *Information about contraception for young people*
  Practical advice for young people about pregnancy and contraception.
  Booklet downloadable from www.avert.org/ypbooks.htm

- *Condoms, Pills and Other Useful Things: a young person's guide to contraception and STIs*
  Booklet downloadable from www.avert.org/ypbooks.htm

- *Nothing But The Facts: condom sense made simple*
  A colourful, pocket-sized leaflet aimed at young people aged 14 and above. It provides a practical guide to condoms, including what they look like, whose responsibility they are, how they are used and where they can be obtained. Available from www.brook.org.uk

- *Nothing But The Facts: hormonal contraception made simple*
  This myth-busting, pocket-sized leaflet presents the facts on different forms of hormonal contraception so young people can make up their own minds. It is aimed at young people aged 14 and above and provides guidance on where to go for expert advice and what to do if things go wrong. Available from www.brook.org.uk

- *Nothing But The Facts: contraception made simple*
  Aimed at young people aged 14 and above, this pocket-sized leaflet provides information on the full range of contraception available for both sexes. A comprehensive list of what is on offer will enable young people to make informed choices when the time comes, as well as know what to do if things go wrong. Available from www.brook.org.uk

- www.learn.co.uk
  Online materials for lesson planning and private study. Provided by *The Guardian*, it is curriculum based and hence has clear guidance on the level of detail required for each age group.

- www.avert.org
  Avert is an international HIV and AIDS charity. The website includes details of contraceptive methods and has some good interactive quizzes on condom use and pregnancy. These quizzes can be printed.

- www.brook.org.uk
  Brook offers free and confidential sexual health advice and contraception to young people up to the age of 25. The website includes simple yet detailed summaries of contraceptive methods.

- www.likeitis.org.uk
  Likeitis gives young people access to information about all aspects of sex education and teenage life. Topics on the likeitis site include: teenage pregnancy, help and advice, periods, lovebugs (sexually transmitted infections), sex, peer pressure, sexuality, contraception, emergency contraception and puberty. Likeitis is part of Marie Stopes International.

- www.wiredforhealth.gov.uk
  Wired for Health is a series of websites managed by the Health Development Agency on behalf of the Department of Health and the Department for Education and Skills.
      Health information that relates to the National Curriculum and the National Healthy School Standard is provided for a range of audiences (*see* Chapter 10 for further details).

- www.mindbodysoul.gov.uk
  Mind, Body and Soul is for 14–16 year-olds (Key Stage 4) and includes an interactive and informative sexual health section.

For professionals

- Everett S (2000) *Handbook of Contraception and Family Planning.* Ballière-Tindall, Edinburgh.
- Guillebaud J (2003) *Contraception: your questions answered.* Churchill Livingstone, London.
- Guillebaud J (2003) *Contraception Today.* Taylor and Francis, London.
- Wilkinson C and Szarewski A (2003) *Contraceptive Dilemmas.* Altman, St Albans.

CHAPTER 6

Young people and sexual health

The prevalence of sexually transmitted infections (STIs) is increasing in the teenage group. Health professionals should be aware of general risk factors pertaining to sexual health and know the local services where young people can obtain sexual health advice and screening. This chapter gives an overview of the current statistics regarding young people's sexual health and explores how their sexual health can be promoted. A broad approach to sexual health screening that can be used by all health professionals who come into contact with young people is set out. The usual routine at a sexual health clinic is described, including the tests performed and the professionals a young person might meet. If professionals working with young people are aware of what happens at these clinics they can help to remove any misconceptions or fears. Finally, some sexual health myths are examined.

Sexually active young people are vulnerable to STIs and, as mentioned above, prevalence amongst young people is increasing: 20–30% of teenage females diagnosed with an STI have another within 18 months.[1] (*See* Chapter 7 for descriptions of individual STIs.)

The consequences of infection with an STI vary according to the infection. They can include increased risk of cervical cancer, pelvic inflammatory disease (PID), ectopic pregnancy and infertility. With acquired immunodeficiency syndrome (AIDS), the individual is susceptible to opportunistic infections and will ultimately die. The consequences of STIs can be worse for teenagers as they tend to present late for treatment, have a poor knowledge of STIs and have unrealistic perceptions of their risks.[2]

Research has shown that there are certain risk factors for contracting STIs (*see* Box 6.1).[1] Professionals who work with young people can use these as a guide to identify young people who are at particular risk. They can then direct health promotion counselling towards improving knowledge, safe sex and accessing contraception and sexual health services.

Box 6.1   Risk factors for STIs[1]

- Male sex
- Young age
- Early age at first intercourse
- Number of partners

- Ethnic group (high rates amongst Afro-Caribbeans, low amongst Asians)
- Failure to use barrier method of contraception
- Low knowledge levels leading to poor perception of risk
- Previous STI
- Male homosexuality
- Attendance at a sexual health clinic

What is sexual health?

The Family Planning Association describes sexual health as 'the capacity and freedom to enjoy and express sexuality without exploitation, oppression, physical or emotional harm'.[3]

The Government's National Strategy for Sexual Health and HIV adds that it is society's duty to inform people of knowledge required for sexual health and to protect their rights to sexual fulfilment:[4]

> Sexual health is an important part of physical and mental health. It is a key part of our identity as human beings together with the fundamental human right to privacy, a family life and living free from discrimination. Essential elements of good sexual health are equitable relationships and sexual fulfilment with access to information and services to avoid the risk of unintended pregnancy, illness or disease.

The National Strategy for Sexual Health and HIV focuses on improving people's sexual health through improving information giving and services. In summary, the goals outlined in the strategy are:[4]

- to reduce unintended pregnancy rates
- to reduce the transmission of STIs and HIV (human immunodeficiency virus)
- to reduce the prevalence of undiagnosed STIs and HIV
- to reduce the stigma associated with STIs and HIV
- to improve health and social care for people living with HIV.

Some of the recommended actions to achieve these goals are: a national information campaign; improving the quality of helplines; improving education about sex and relationships; prevention for groups at special risk, e.g. drug users, young offenders, gay men, etc.; a national chlamydia screening programme (see Box 6.2); developing one-stop shops where clients can obtain advice, contraceptive and GUM services on a single site.

Box 6.2   Chlamydia Screening Programme

The NHS Plan, introduced in 2000, included a commitment to improving the prevention of ill health and providing screening programmes where effective.[5] Chlamydia is a serious problem: around 9% of sexually active young women are likely to be infected and around 70% of infections are asymptomatic. The consequences of untreated infection can be serious, and include PID and subsequent infertility.[6]

The Department of Health carried out chlamydia screening pilots in Portsmouth and the Wirral between September 1999 and August 2000. These focused on women aged 16–24 as they are more likely to attend health-care settings and the consequences of infection are more serious for women than men.

The early indications are that these programmes are acceptable to both the public and professionals and the National Strategy for Sexual Health and HIV has recommended a phased national implementation of chlamydia screening. The first phase is now under way in England and covers ten primary care trust areas and up to 400 individual testing sites.

Sexual health and young people

It is during the teenage years that sexual identity becomes important to a young person. As discussed in Chapter 1, physically and physiologically the young person is experiencing many changes in body structure and hormone levels and psychologically they are trying to establish a sexual identity. This period may be confusing for the young person and often sexual contact is unplanned.

Adolescents may be well informed about safe sex practices but do not necessarily use the information they have. The circumstances at the time of the sexual encounter (e.g. condom availability) and the ability of the couple to communicate and negotiate contraception use can influence choices. In a UK study, 89% of teenagers acknowledged that having sex without using condoms put them at risk of HIV/AIDS but 16% would still have unprotected intercourse if the opportunity arose. For teenage boys this figure was 23%, suggesting that they are more likely to take risks than girls.[7]

Contraception provision: has this caused STIs to increase in young people?

Recent research has highlighted a worrying correlation between an increase in contraception provision and a rise in STIs in young people.[8] Naturally, this has caused a great furore in the Press, who have suggested that the whole Teenage Pregnancy Strategy has been a waste of time. But before all professionals working in this area become despondent, a closer look at the research can help refine practice rather than abandon it.

The paper by David Paton, Professor of Industrial Economics at Nottingham University Business School, considers the behavioural response of adolescents to contraception provision from an economics angle.[8] Do young people make a rational choice between sexual activity and abstention based on the expected utility of each choice (weighing up the pros and cons of sexual activity); or is sexual activity in this age group random, where the young people either do not have the information they require to make safe choices regarding sexual activity or, if they do, they cannot apply the information effectively?

Policy to date, namely the Teenage Pregnancy Strategy, has worked on the principle that young people's sexual activity is of the random decision-making model. If a sexually active adolescent moves from not using contraception to using a barrier method, pregnancy rates and STI rates will decrease. If a sexually active adolescent moves from not using contraception to a non-barrier method there will be a reduction in pregnancy rates and no change in STI rates. Thus the increased availability of contraception provision should improve pregnancy and STI rates.

The increased availability of hormonal emergency contraception, according to the random decision-making model, will reduce pregnancy and not effect any change in STI rates.

However, if young people are making a rational choice to have sex based on the perceived outcomes and their cost (pregnancy and STIs) there are two possible outcomes: an increase in availability of family planning will lead to those who choose sex being more likely to use some form of contraception, lowering the probability of pregnancy; yet lowering the cost of sexual activity in relation to abstinence will mean some young people who previously chose abstinence will now choose sex, and some of these will become pregnant due to the failure or misuse of the contraceptive method.

A straightforward prediction of pregnancy or STI rates is not possible with the rational decision-making model: pregnancy rates may increase, decrease or remain static; and with more young people becoming sexually active, depending on their choice of contraceptive method, infection rates will either remain the same or increase.

The availability of hormonal emergency contraception again reduces the cost of sexual activity and, in Paton's words, 'weakens a woman's bargaining power at the time when effective decisions over sexual activity are taken';[8] therefore the reduction in cost would be predicted to result in an increase in STI rates.

David Paton's research found that a 23% increase in clinic sessions 'led to' a 1.45% increase in STI rates. These results came from data gathered over a four-year period from 1999 to 2002, which included the year before the Teenage Pregnancy Strategy, the year of its implementation and two subsequent years. This supports Government data which states that sexual activity amongst 16–19 year-olds has risen by 12%, conception rates have fallen by 3.5% and STI rates have increased by 15.8%. This is alongside a rise in clinic sessions offered from 27 075 to 33 369.[8] Therefore as STI rates are increasing, it would suggest that young people are making a rational decision to have sex and that we, by making contraception more easily available, are encouraging young people to have sex.

So should we abandon current practice and go back to the drawing board on tackling teenage pregnancy and STIs? Should we go the way of America and focus on abstention to the exclusion of giving information on accessing and using contraception and practising safe sex? Should we focus on the cost of sexual activity with scare-tactic messages of infertility from STIs and that all condoms have holes in them?[9] This doesn't appear to be effective either as the United States has higher teenage pregnancy rates than the UK.

What is required is a re-examination of practice. Some young people will be making 'random decisions' to enter into a sexual relationship and increased availability of contraception will prevent pregnancy. Yet for those who are being encouraged to be sexually active (making a rational decision based on the reduced cost to self), we should go back to the original research that shows exposure to a comprehensive sex and relationships programme delays first sex and improves safe sex practice.[1] The emphasis needs to be placed on 'comprehensive'. The value of abstention should be presented alongside factual information on using and accessing contraceptive methods, with emphasis on condom use to prevent STIs.

Health promotion programmes – outreach in schools and youth groups, the sex and relationships education (SRE) curriculum – are difficult to measure, so it has been more appealing to set up clinics where numbers of attendances and outcomes can be crunched. Even within health promotion programmes it is easier to present a session on contraceptive methods or the details of STIs rather than grapple with negotiation skills and self-esteem. 'Comprehensive' sexual health promotion programmes are being implemented in youth settings, and these are increasingly being supported and underpinned by Government policy (SRE curriculum, Healthy School Standard) and research (*see* the extensive publications by the National Children's Bureau, fpa and Brook). It can be an uphill struggle as we are often contradicting the all-pervasive message in the media and fashion that sex is good and everybody is doing it. It takes time to build self-esteem, to practise negotiation and decision-making skills, but in time we will see the fruits of our labour.

Understanding young people's sexual behaviour requires a shift away from simple concepts of illness/pregnancy avoidance towards a much greater appreciation of issues such as power between individuals, constraints and social reputation. There may also be other factors influencing a young person's ability to make reasoned decisions such as alcohol or drug intoxication and peer pressure.

Young people are increasingly using drugs and alcohol and at younger ages (*see* Chapter 1). A survey by the Health Education Authority looking at young people and sexual intercourse under the influence of drugs and/or alcohol showed that:[10]

- one in five had had sex they later regretted
- one in seven had had unsafe sex
- one in ten had been unable to remember whether they had had sex the night before.

The use of drugs and alcohol inhibits a young person's ability to make informed decisions about sexual intercourse.

Peer pressure can also be an influential factor over young people's sexual activity. The same survey found that for young people aged 14 and 15, friends were as influential as a source of information about sex as school.[10] This information is not always reliable and may perpetuate myths around sex and contraception. There is a lot of talk about sex amongst young people; individuals may feel they are the only ones not to have had sex and may enter into an early sexual relationship as a result. Also, within a relationship a young person may not have the self-esteem and negotiation skills to refuse sex if they do not feel ready (*see* Chapter 1).

Improving sexual health

It is vital to provide comprehensive sex and relationships education to improve a young person's ability to negotiate levels of intimacy and contraception use within a relationship, and to provide knowledge of STIs, contraceptive choices and where to access services. In addition there should be STI diagnosis and treatment centres and contraception provision that are accessible to young people.

Historically there have been three main aspects to sexual health services for young people: sex education in schools, contraceptive advice and provision (usually in GP surgeries and family planning clinics), and diagnosis and treatment of STIs in genito-urinary medicine (GUM) clinics. Increasingly, new and innovative methods of reaching young people are being developed; there has been great improvement in the SRE curriculum in schools; sexual health clinics specifically for young people are being set up and mainstream provision is improving sexual health services for young people.

SRE and abstinence campaigns

Sex and relationships education is essential if young people are to have the information required to make informed decisions regarding their sexual health. When consulted, young people frequently say that SRE in school was too little too late and that it only addressed the mechanics of sex.[11] Adults are often concerned that introducing sex education too early may encourage young people to have sex sooner. Research has indicated that the opposite is true: well-informed young people delay first sex and when they do have sexual intercourse they are more likely to use a condom.[11] (Chapter 10 looks at how to support parents in communicating with their teenagers and explores how to deliver effective SRE in school and youth settings.)

Campaigns to promote abstinence, such as the 'True Love Waits' movement in America, have a big following. It has yet to be replicated in England on such a scale. It is beneficial if young people delay sexual intercourse in that they are less likely to contract STIs, become pregnant or suffer the psychological damage of breakdown in relationships. However, the abstinence message often omits to give any information on sexual health and contraception; or perpetuates false information such as all condoms have holes in them and therefore do not protect against pregnancy and STIs.[12] Therefore if young people who have opted into this movement do become sexually active, they are far less likely to use contraception than other teens – partly because they spent those months denying that they would ever need it – and so increase their risks of pregnancy and disease.[12] What we *can* learn from abstinence education programmes is that teaching young people techniques to resist pressure to have sex is a way of empowering them. Teaching this skill would fit within the directives of SRE by encouraging respect for self and others.

For effective SRE a combination of approaches is needed: motivating young people to adopt abstinence and delay first intercourse and – for those who are or become sexually active – giving them the negotiation skills and knowledge to protect against unwanted pregnancies and disease.

Sexual health and contraception services

Sexual health and contraception services should be developed in the light of a local needs assessment that incorporates provider and client views. Confidentiality and easy access to services should be ensured. In 1996, the Health Education Authority published a guide to good practice in contraception services for young people. The following characteristics of good practice were identified:[13]

- young people should have a choice of services; there should be a range of service options for young people based in a variety of locations: community, clinic, school, college, town centre
- services should integrate contraceptive and GUM services, and should link with agencies concerned with more general aspects of young people's health
- services should be accessible; for example, with extended opening hours
- young men should be targeted with separate clinic provision
- staff should be committed to working with young people; they should have an understanding of the issues affecting young people and experience of working in non-traditional settings.

Similar points are reiterated in the National Strategy for Sexual Health and HIV.[4]

The venue is important; a service's decor and ambiance should be welcoming to young people (*see* Chapter 9 for further information regarding issues to consider when setting up a young person's clinic). Consideration should be given to how services will meet the needs of different target groups, e.g. ethnic groups, young people with a disability, etc. Traditional names for sexual health services such as 'family planning' or 'genito-urinary' clinics are off-putting for young people and less formal titles are preferred.

Partnership working is essential in providing effective, accessible and holistic services; through drawing on a range of expertise and experience, partnerships can provide access routes to services which more traditional approaches cannot. For example, health professionals teamed up with the youth service in Chester-le-Street to provide a weekly sexual health advisory and contraception service at the youth club disco (*see* Box 6.3).[14] (Working in partnership will be discussed in more detail in Chapter 9.)

STI screening

All health professionals working with young people can carry out broad sexual health screening. Aside from diagnosis through physiological symptoms, the following are questions that can highlight risk factors and concerns surrounding a young person's sexual health:

Box 6.3   Sexual health clinic for young people at Chester-le-Street Youth Centre[14]

'Teenage Confidential' is a sexual health clinic specifically designed for young people. It is held every Thursday from 6.45pm to 7.45pm.

A young person named the clinic and young people have been extensively consulted in the clinic's design and layout. The clinic has been organised in partnership with the youth centre, that provides a bus to enable young people from surrounding villages to attend a weekly disco.

Services are scarce in the outlying villages. It's a good opportunity for young people who are attending the disco to receive information, advice and contraceptive services in an informal setting.

- What is the young person's knowledge about sexual health? Do they need information regarding safe sex, contraception and STIs?
- Do they understand the risk of STIs and unplanned pregnancy? What is their understanding of how a young woman becomes pregnant?
- Are they engaging in drug and alcohol misuse that may make them more likely to engage in unprotected sexual intercourse?
- Are they being sexually or physically abused? Is sex non-consensual? (If so, it is unlikely they will be able to insist on condom use.)
- How old is their partner? If he or she is significantly older, is it an appropriate relationship?
- Do they have any psychological problems that may make them vulnerable to sexual predators?

If a professional has any concerns about a young person's sexual health, with the young person's agreement they can refer them on to an appropriate service, e.g. contraception, diagnostic screening or counselling. If there are non-clinical concerns they can liaise with other agencies that can support the young person, e.g. social services (if there is a child protection concern), local drug and alcohol support services, youth service or young person's clinic. It is important to have a comprehensive knowledge of local agencies that can support young people.

Sexual health services

There are dedicated departments for sexual health screening in most hospitals and these may have specific young people's clinics; in addition there are increasing numbers of community clinics that offer sexual health screening (*see* Box 6.4), and GP surgeries offer tests for some STIs. All services offer the same degree of confidentiality to young people.

Box 6.4   Choices N4: City and Hackney Young People's Services

This project offers genito-urinary (GU) screening, contraception services and counselling for under-26s on a drop-in basis in a community health centre. It is staffed by three nurses, a health adviser, counsellor, doctor and two reception staff.

This project is part of an overall team that provides:

- a drop-in advisory service in a local college
- an SRE team that supports teachers in the PSE curriculum
- outreach in youth settings
- dedicated young people's contraception clinics in the community
- a GU screening and contraception clinic in the local hospital
- a partnership organisation in a Lesbian, Gay, Bisexual and Transgender drop-in.

Due to the comprehensive outreach and community-based education work carried out by project staff, large numbers of young people access the service for STI check-ups and contraception.

What happens at the sexual health clinic?

Young people are put off by the unknown and benefit from knowing what they are likely to encounter when attending a sexual health clinic. This could be communicated through an informal session with a youth group or school: a representative from the clinic could present a session or offer tours of the clinic. This would be an ideal opportunity for any myths and fears surrounding sexual health to be dispelled and for young people to voice any concerns or questions.

This section briefly describes what happens at the sexual health clinic, the questions that are asked, the professionals that the young people may see and the tests that may be carried out.

Registration

The first step at a sexual health clinic is to fill in a form. For the clinic records a name and date of birth are needed; the clinic will not contact the client's doctor or parents without their permission or knowledge. If the client is under 16, the clinic doctor, health adviser or nurse may recommend they tell their parents (as it is a recommendation by law in the Fraser Guidelines; *see* Chapter 3). Each person is given a card with a clinic number; this should be brought at each visit. It should be possible to request to be seen by someone of a particular gender.

Interview

The young person is then seen by a trained member of staff, who will ask personal questions about their sex life. This 'sexual history' helps decide what investigations (if any) should be done. For example:

- What are your concerns?
- How many people have you had sex with recently?
- What type of sex was it?
- Were your partners male or female?
- Have you had an STI in the past?
- Are you taking any medication?
- Do you have any allergies?

Examination

If the client agrees they will then have some tests and swabs taken. This may be embarrassing and possibly a bit uncomfortable, but the clinic staff are aware of this and will explain what is going on. All treatment is free. Examination and tests will vary according to a person's sex and stated sexual practice. Any question should be answered truthfully so nothing is overlooked. If the young person is unsure why a question is being asked or words are used that they don't understand, a clearer explanation should be given.

Tests *may* include:

- a urine test (it is best not to go to the toilet for two hours before)
- a cervical smear (where cells are taken from the cervix with a spatula; these are put onto a slide and sent to the laboratory for testing. The test checks for cells that may develop into cervical cancer). (*See* Appendix 6 for further details of cervical screening.)
- swabs from the urethra, vagina, cervix, throat and rectum. A speculum is used to hold open the vagina and the doctor or nurse may insert gloved fingers at the same time. They do this to locate the cervix or to check for tenderness. A small tube called a proctoscope may in some cases be inserted into the rectum
- blood test for syphilis.

HIV tests are only done with consent and are not routinely performed. The test for HIV is a blood test.

Diagnosis

The presence of some infections can be detected straight away by what can be seen on examination and looking through a microscope at what has been put on slides from the swabs. Other swabs need to be sent to a laboratory and take several days for the results to become known. A client may be asked to return for further tests at the end of a specified time period before a full diagnosis can be made. For example, HIV and syphilis take up to three months after infection to show up on a blood test. A full explanation should be given of test results and relevant leaflets supplied to back up any advice given.

Treatment

Treatment is free and often given straight away. A full course of antibiotics should be taken even if the symptoms clear before they are finished.

Who will you see?

Doctor and nurse

A doctor or a nurse will do the interview at the beginning and take the swabs and blood. If you need any treatment they will also explain why and what should be taken.

Health adviser

Most clinics have a health adviser who can spend time helping clients better understand what is going on. There may be personal issues a client would like to talk through; for example, they can help when working out what to do about current or previous partners who may need to be examined or treated.

When a person is found to have an STI, it is important to find out who else might have it. This is so those people can be tested and treated. Often they do not know they have an STI. Treating these people prevents disease and future complications. The process is called 'partner notification'. This is important in helping to control the spread of infections.

Sexual health myths

'With advances in medicine, there is no need to worry about sexually transmitted infections. It only takes a course of antibiotics and you are fine, anyway!'

Most STIs can be completely cured if they are caught at an early stage, and the treatment can be as simple as a course of antibiotics. This is one of the reasons why it's a good idea to be tested regularly, and why you should go immediately to a health professional if you have any concerns about an STI.
    However:

- If left untreated, STIs can pose a long-term risk to your health and fertility. Chlamydia and gonorrhoea can both lead to PID if they are not treated. This can lead to long-term pelvic pain, blocked uterine tubes, infertility and ectopic pregnancy in women; and pain and inflammation of the testicles and the prostate gland in men.
- Genital warts and genital herpes are two common viral infections; antibiotics, that can only treat bacterial infections, will not treat them. Acute occurrences can be treated with antiviral medications, but both conditions can come back.
- Although antiretroviral drugs have been developed to slow the progression of HIV to AIDS, there is still no cure.

'Condoms protect against all STIs.'

Using a condom for oral, anal and vaginal sex is a good protection against most STIs. However, condoms don't necessarily protect against the transmission of genital warts or herpes through skin-to-skin contact.

'Anyone infected with an STI will have obvious symptoms such as a rash or discharge.'

There are many potential signs of an STI. These include:

- itching around the genitals or anus
- burning or pain when you urinate
- bleeding and pain during or after sex
- rashes, blisters or bumps around the genitals or anus
- unusual discharge from the penis or vagina.

However, many STIs have no symptoms at all. (*See* Chapter 7 for details on STIs.)

References

1   Social Exclusion Unit (1999) *Teenage Pregnancy Strategy*. HMSO, London.
2   Lindsay J (2001) *Providing Sexual Health to Teenagers*. North and South Islington Primary Care Trust, London.

3   www.fpa.org.uk/news/docs/sexoffs (2003)
4   Department of Health (2001) *National Strategy for Sexual Health and HIV.* HMSO, London.
5   Department of Health (2000) *The NHS Plan.* HMSO, London.
6   National Health Service (2003) *Chlamydia Infection.* National electronic Library for Health. www.nelh.nhs.uk/screening/adult_pps/chlamydia.html
7   Johnson A, Wadsworth J, Wellings K *et al.* (1994) *Sexual Attitudes and Lifestyles.* Blackwell Scientific Publications, London.
8   Paton D (2004) *Random Behaviour or Rational Choice? Family Planning, Teenage Pregnancy and STIs.* Presented at the Royal Economic Society Conference, Swansea.
9   www.channel4.com (2004) *Texas Teenage Virgins.*
10 Health Education Authority (1998) *Unintended Teenage Conceptions.* HEA, London.
11 Save the Children (2002) *Get Real: providing dedicated sexual health services for young people.* Save the Children, London.
12 Swan C, Bowe K, McCormick G *et al.* (2003) *Teenage Pregnancy and Parenthood: a review of reviews.* Evidence Briefing. www.hda-online.org.uk/documents/teenpreg_evidence_briefing.pdf
13 Aggleton P, Baldo M and Slutkin G (1996) *Promoting Young People's Sexual Health: a compendium of family planning provision for young people.* Health Education Authority, London.
14 Watson G (2003) *News Archive: new sexual health clinic for young people at Chester-le-Street Youth Centre.* www.health-promotion.org.uk/resources

Resources

* Save the Children (2002) *Get Real: providing dedicated sexual health services for young people.* Save the Children, London.
  Following research into sexual health services for young people this document seeks to support policy makers, service commissioners and practitioners by providing guidance on what works and why from a young person's point of view. Available from Save the Children, c/o Pymbridge Distributors Ltd, Estover Road, Plymouth PL6 7PY.

* Sexual Health Forum (2001) *Working with Young People in Sexual Health Settings: a provider's guide.* Factsheet 25. National Children's Bureau, London. www.ncb.org.uk/sexed.htm
  Factsheet giving guidance on developing appropriate, sensitive sexual health services that are young people-friendly.

* Faculty of Family Planning and Reproductive Health Care (2003) *Faculty of Family Planning and Reproductive Health Care of the Royal College of Obstetricians and Gynaecologists Service Standards for Sexual Health Services.* RCOG, London. www.ffprhc.org.uk/Service%Standards%20-%20FINAL2.pdf

- www.teenagepregnancyunit.gov.uk
  Guidance for youth workers on providing information and referring young people to contraceptive and sexual health services.

- www.ruthinking.co.uk
  A website run by Sexwise, an independent charity, offering information and advice about sex, relationships, emergency help and local services. Sexwise also runs a free, confidential helpline on sex, relationships and contraception. Tel: 0800 28 29 30.

- www.mindbodysoul.gov.uk
  A site developed by the Department of Health. Designed for Key Stage 4 pupils (aged 14–16), it covers a variety of health topics. The Sexual Health option provides information and advice on a range of topics as well as links to other related sites. Other options include: Choices; Contraception; STIs; Help and Support; Common Questions; Growing and Changing; Friendships and Relationships; Sexuality; Is Everybody Doing It?

- www.lovelife.uk.com/clinics
  A directory to UK young people's sexual health clinics.

- *Nothing But The Facts: safer sex made simple*
  This leaflet is aimed at young people aged 14 and above. It describes what constitutes safer sex and how to avoid STIs as well as pregnancy.
  www.brook.org.uk

CHAPTER 7

Young people and sexually transmitted infections

This chapter describes the more common sexually transmitted infections, such as chlamydia, gonorrhoea, genital warts and herpes, outlining their symptoms, how they are transmitted and the treatment available. Books with greater detail are available and a selection is listed in the resources section at the end of the chapter, together with some excellent websites that communicate the facts about STIs through interactive games and visuals.

National guidelines have been produced on the management of suspected STIs in children and young people. It is recommended that the reader check the Association for Genito-Urinary Medicine website to keep up to date with any changes in recommended practice (www.agum.org.uk/guidelines.htm).

Chlamydia

Chlamydia is the most common STI in the UK. Between 2001 and 2002 there was a 14% rise in the number of cases of chlamydia diagnosed in sexual health clinics; a rise of 15% in men and 13% in women. The number of cases has risen steadily since the mid 1990s and more than doubled from around 34 100 cases diagnosed in 1996 to just under 81 700 in 2002.[1]

The highest rates are seen in young people, especially women under 25 years. In 2002, 16–19 year-old females had the highest chlamydia rate at 1201 per 100 000 females seen at clinics; a diagnostic rate equivalent to almost 1%. Among men, the highest rate was for those aged 20–24 at 837 per 100 000.[1]

Genital chlamydial infection is an important reproductive health problem, as 10–30% of infected women develop pelvic inflammatory disease (PID).[1]

Symptoms

The majority of women who are infected with chlamydia will not have symptoms, but some may notice:

- increased vaginal discharge
- frequent or painful urination
- lower abdominal pain
- pain during sex
- irregular periods.

Men are more likely to notice symptoms, but some may not have any. They may experience:

- discharge from the penis
- pain/burning on urination.

Sometimes the eyes can become infected with chlamydia; both men and women can experience painful swelling and irritation of the eyes.

Transmission

Chlamydia can be transmitted in the following ways:

- penetrative sex (where the penis enters the vagina, mouth or anus)
- mother to baby during birth
- occasionally by transferring the infection on fingers from the genitals to the eyes.

Diagnosis and treatment

Samples will be taken from areas that may be infected such as the vagina and cervix in women, or the urethra in men, and sent to a laboratory for testing. A urine sample may also be taken. The results are usually available within a week. If the test is positive, the treatment for chlamydia is a simple course of antibiotics.

Long-term effects

In women, if left untreated, chlamydia can lead to PID, fertility problems, ectopic pregnancy, reactive arthritis, Bartholin's abscess and chronic pelvic pain. For men there can be complications such as sub-fertility, epididymitis, epididymo-orchitis and reactive arthritis.

Gonorrhoea

Gonorrhoea is the second most common STI. In 2002 there were 24 953 infections diagnosed in sexual health clinics; a 9% increase from 2001. Young people are most commonly infected.

The number of new cases of gonorrhoea diagnosed in sexual health clinics has risen every year since 1995. Between 1998 and 1999, the number of cases in England and Wales rose by 25%, and between 1999 and 2000 there was a further 27% increase. Although men were much more likely than women to be diagnosed with gonorrhoea, the rise in incidence occurred in both sexes. The biggest rises have occurred amongst teenagers: between 1995 and 2000 the number of cases of gonorrhoea amongst young people aged 19 and under more than doubled.[2]

Signs and symptoms

It is possible to be infected with gonorrhoea and not have symptoms. Men are far more likely to notice symptoms than women.

Symptoms in women may include:

- a change in vaginal discharge. This may increase, change to a yellow or green-ish colour and develop a strong smell
- a pain or burning sensation when passing urine
- irritation of and/or discharge from the anus.

Symptoms in men may include:

- a yellow or white discharge from the penis
- irritation of and/or discharge from the anus
- inflammation of the testicles and prostate gland.

Transmission

Gonorrhoea is passed on through:

- penetrative sex

and less often by:

- inserting your fingers into an infected vagina, anus or mouth and then putting them into your own without washing your hands in between
- sharing vibrators or other sex toys.

Diagnosis and treatment

Samples are taken, using a cotton wool or spongy swab, from any area that may be infected – the cervix, urethra, anus or throat. A sample of urine may also be taken. Samples taken are looked at under a microscope and it may be possible to make a diagnosis immediately. A second sample is sent to a laboratory for diagnosis or confirmation and results are available within a week. If the tests are positive, antibiotics can be given.

Long-term effects

If left untreated, gonorrhoea can lead to PID in women. This can cause fever, pain and lead to infertility or ectopic pregnancy.

A woman can pass gonorrhoea on to her baby if she is infected when the baby is born.

In men, gonorrhoea can cause inflammation of the testicles and the prostate gland, which causes pain. Without treatment the urethra may become narrower.

Genital warts

Anogenital warts (first attack) is the most common viral STI diagnosed in sexual health clinics, comprising 10% (69 449 of 677 225) of all diagnoses in 2002.

Between 1972 and 2002, the number of all genital warts diagnoses (first episode, recurrent and re-registered cases) increased more than six- and tenfold in men and women, respectively. These rises may reflect increased incidence of infection, greater public awareness and/or improved diagnostic sensitivity.

For males, highest rates of new cases are found in 20–24 year-olds (776/100 000) and for females in 16–19 year-olds (682/100 000); 29% of diagnoses amongst females were seen in those under 20 years of age. (This compares to 9% in males.)[1]

Signs and symptoms

- Pinkish/white small lumps or larger cauliflower-shaped lumps on the genital area.
- Warts on the vulva, penis, scrotum or anus, in the vagina and on the cervix.
- It usually takes one to three months from infection for the warts to appear.
- They may itch but are usually painless.
- Not everyone who comes into contact with the virus will develop warts.

Transmission

Warts are spread through skin-to-skin contact and can therefore be caught through genital contact as well as sexual intercourse.

Diagnosis and treatment

A doctor or nurse can usually diagnose genital warts by looking. A test may be performed by applying a solution to the outside of the genital area. This turns any warts white. An internal examination may be carried out to check for warts in the vagina or anus.

A common treatment for genital warts is to paint on a brown liquid called podophyllin. They can also be treated by freezing or laser treatment.

A client diagnosed with genital warts should:

- keep the genital area clean and dry
- not use scented soaps, bath oils or vaginal deodorants
- use condoms when having sex (these will protect against warts only if they cover the affected area).

Long-term effects

Most people will have a recurrence of warts that will need further treatment. Some types of the wart virus may be linked to changes in cervical cells that can lead to cervical cancer. It is important that all women over 25 years of age have a regular cervical smear test (*see* Appendix 6).

Genital herpes

In 2002, 18 388 men and women attended sexual health clinics in England, Wales and Northern Ireland with first-attack genital herpes simplex virus (HSV). The prevalence of HSV infection increases with increasing age. Less than 5% of adolescents have genital herpes, but this figure more than doubles in the 20–24 age group, where rates of diagnosis are highest.[1]

Signs and symptoms

Both men and women may have one or more symptoms, including:

- itching or tingling sensation in the genital or anal area
- small fluid-filled blisters in the genital or anal area. These burst and leave small sores that can be painful. In time they dry out, scab over and heal. The first infection can take between two and four weeks to heal
- pain when passing urine, if it passes over any of the open sores
- a flu-like illness, backache, headache, swollen glands or fever. (At this time the virus is highly infectious.)

Recurrent infections are usually milder. The sores are fewer, smaller, less painful and heal more quickly.

Transmission

HSV is passed on through direct contact with an infected person. The virus affects the areas where it enters the body. This can be by:

- kissing (mouth to mouth)
- penetrative sex (when the penis enters the vagina, mouth or anus)
- oral sex (from mouth to the genitals and vice versa).

Diagnosis and treatment

A clinical examination of the genital area is carried out by a doctor or a nurse. A sample is taken, using a cotton wool or spongy swab, from any visible sores. Samples are then sent to a laboratory for testing and the results should be available within two weeks.

Tablets can reduce the severity of the infection; these are only effective when taken within 72 hours of the start of the symptoms. A cream is available to control the symptoms. Recurrent infections may not need treatment.

During an episode of herpes, the blisters and sores are highly infectious and the virus can be passed on to others by direct contact. To prevent this from happening the following should be avoided:

- kissing when there are cold sores around the mouth
- oral sex when there are mouth or genital sores
- any genital or anal contact, even with a condom or dental dam, when there are genital sores
- sharing towels and face flannels.

Long-term effects

Having herpes does not affect a woman's ability to become pregnant, but if herpes occurs in the first three months of pregnancy there is a small risk of miscarriage.[3] If an individual has an episode of herpes when the baby is due, they may be advised to have a Caesarean delivery to reduce the risk of infecting the baby.

Other common STIs are non-specific urethritis in men and *Trichomonas vaginalis*. Syphilis is generally uncommon although there are certain geographical pockets where resurgences are occurring.

Non-specific urethritis (NSU)

Non-specific urethritis only affects men. Chlamydia is the most common cause of NSU, accounting for 30–50% of cases. Trichomonas vaginitis has been reported in 1–17% of NSU cases. Infections from the *Ureaplasma urealyticum* and *Mycoplasma genitalium* species account for 10% and 20% of cases, respectively. Other infections such as HSV, thrush and bacterial urinary tract infections (UTIs) only account for a small proportion of cases. There is also a possible association with bacterial vaginosis. Between 20% and 30% of NSU cases have no organism detected. The infection that causes NSU could potentially cause genital tract inflammation and PID in women.[4]

Signs and symptoms

These may include inflammation of a man's urethra, causing pain or burning when passing urine, discharge from the penis and frequent urination.

Transmission

Several different types of infection can cause NSU; most often transmitted through penetrative sex, it can occur rarely through friction during sex, allergy or excess alcohol.

Diagnosis and treatment

A doctor or nurse may carry out a physical examination of the genital area and swabs are taken from the penis or urethra; these are then examined under the microscope. Swabs are sent for culture and a urine sample is taken. NSU is easily treated with antibiotics.

Long-term effects

NSU rarely reappears. Serious complications can be inflammation of the testicles and reduced fertility.

Trichomonas vaginalis (TV)

In 1997, sexual health clinics in the UK reported over 5600 cases of TV in women and 250 cases in men. Prevalence is highest in those aged 20–45 years. TV is identified in 30–40% of male sexual partners of infected women.[5]

Signs and symptoms

Often TV is asymptomatic, but in both men and women there can be discharge, genital soreness, pain when passing urine and pain during sex.

Diagnosis and treatment

Swabs from the urethra or vagina and urine samples are taken; swabs are examined under the microscope and cultured. TV is easily treated with antibiotics.

Long-term effects

Complications associated with TV are rare; if a woman is infected when she gives birth, she may pass it on to a female child.[6]

Syphilis

From 1998 to 1999, diagnoses of syphilis in the UK rose by 58% amongst men and 27% amongst women (*see* Table 7.1).[7] Outbreaks have been noted in the following cities: Bristol, London, Manchester, Brighton, Hove, Dublin and Peterborough. Most cases have been acquired in the UK and are linked through sexual and social networks. Outbreaks have been linked to sex workers, drug users, both homosexual and heterosexual practice, and oral sex. Syphilis appears to facilitate HIV transmission and its progression may be more rapid in people who are HIV-positive.[8]

Table 7.1   Syphilis cases in the UK[7]

Year	No. of cases
1996	122
1997	151
1998	132
1999	215
2000	327
2001	734
2002	1193
% change between 2001 and 2002	63%
% change between 1996 and 2002	878%

Signs and symptoms

Syphilis has three stages:

- primary stage symptoms – sores can develop where bacteria entered the body
- secondary stage symptoms – a rash, warty growths on the genitals and a flu-like illness may develop
- latent stage symptoms – if left untreated, over time syphilis can lead to heart, joint and nervous system damage.

Transmission

Syphilis can be passed on during primary or secondary stages through:

- oral, vaginal or anal sex
- skin contact with any sores or rashes
- from a mother to unborn child.

It is not usually infectious during the latent stage.

Diagnosis and treatment

Blood will be taken and swabs for any sores. A visual examination will be carried out. Syphilis is easily treated by a two-week course of penicillin injections and/or antibiotic tablets or capsules.

If a person is in the early infectious stages of syphilis, oral, vaginal or anal sex is not recommended. Nor is any kind of sex recommended that involves contact between two people and any sores or rashes they may have, until the treatment is completed. Once the treatment is completed they will be required to attend the clinic at regular intervals for blood tests.

Long-term effects

In pregnancy, syphilis can cause miscarriage or stillbirth and be passed from mother to unborn child in the womb.[9] Left untreated, syphilis can cause heart, joint and nervous system damage.[10]

Thrush, bacterial vaginosis and cystitis

Thrush, bacterial vaginosis and cystitis are not necessarily sexually transmitted. Whilst they can occur through other means independently of sexual intercourse, they are included here as they can be precipitated by sex. Sexual intercourse can alter the pH of the vagina where thrush and bacterial vaginosis can colonise. Sex can also introduce bacteria to the urethra in men and women, causing cystitis.

Thrush

Thrush is caused by a yeast that normally lives harmlessly on the skin, or in the mouth, gut and vagina, without causing any problems. Usually it is kept in check by harmless bacteria. Occasionally conditions change and the yeast increases rapidly, causing symptoms.

Between 1990 and 2000, thrush diagnosis in females increased by 34% from 50 945 to 68 298. Despite this increase, the number of attendances for thrush as a proportion of all sexual health clinic attendances fell from 17% in 1990 to 11% in 2000. In 1999, highest rates of diagnosis amongst females were seen in the London (628 per 100 000) and Eastern (263 per 100 000) regions.[1]

Sexual transmission is thought to play a limited part in the epidemiology of thrush. Systemic antibiotic therapy for other conditions may cause thrush to develop; the rise in diagnoses could reflect increased antibiotic use as well as increased sexual health clinic attendance.

Signs and symptoms

Symptoms in women may include:

- itching, soreness and redness around the vagina, vulva or anus
- a thick, white discharge from the vagina that looks like cottage cheese and smells yeasty
- a swollen vulva
- pain during sex
- pain when passing urine.

Symptoms in men may include:

- irritation, burning or itching under the foreskin or on the tip of the penis
- a redness, or red patches, under the foreskin or on the tip of the penis
- a thick, cheesy discharge under the foreskin
- difficulty in pulling back the foreskin
- a slight discharge from the urethra
- discomfort when passing urine.

How thrush develops

There is an increased chance of developing thrush with the following:

- wearing lycra shorts or tight nylon clothes
- taking certain antibiotics
- using too much vaginal deodorant or perfumed bubble bath, causing irritation
- having sex with someone who has a thrush infection
- diabetes.

Any man can develop thrush, but it is more likely in uncircumcised men, who should wash under their foreskins as part of their daily hygiene routine.

Diagnosis and treatment
Thrush is diagnosed by:

- an examination of the genital area by a doctor or nurse
- samples are taken using swabs from anywhere you may have thrush for close examination under a microscope.

A cream is applied to the external genital area and women may be given pessaries to insert into the vagina with an applicator. Oral anti-thrush tablets are also available.

Bacterial vaginosis

Bacterial vaginosis (BV) is a common infection of the vagina. It is the most common cause of abnormal vaginal discharge in women of child-bearing age, and is twice as common as vaginal thrush.

BV is one of the most common reasons for attendance at sexual health clinics, accounting for 9% of female attendances in 2000. Between 1990 and 2000, diagnosis of BV increased by 129% from 27 252 to 62 475. Highest rates were seen in the London (64 per 100 000 population) and Trent (194 per 100 000 population) regions. This is probably a conservative number as 50% of infections are asymptomatic. A prevalence of 12% has been reported by antenatal clinics and 28% by termination of pregnancy clinics, and a recent study in general practice reported a 9% prevalence.[11]

Signs and symptoms
Vaginal discharge; white-grey in colour and fishy smelling.

Diagnosis and treatment
BV is not caused by a single bacterium, but an overgrowth of various bacteria in the vagina. Nor is it caused by poor hygiene; in fact excessive washing of the vagina may alter the normal balance of the bacteria, thus making BV more likely to develop. A nurse or doctor will take a vaginal swab for examination under the microscope and observe the vaginal area for discharge and characteristic smell.

BV can be easily treated with antibiotics. To prevent recurrences the following are also recommended:

- no vaginal douching
- no added bath oils, detergents or bubble bath to bath water
- do not wash around the vaginal area too often.

Complications
While BV is predominantly a vaginal infection, there is concern that it could cause PID under certain circumstances, e.g. following surgical procedures such as termination of pregnancy and hysterectomy. It can cause problems in pregnancy: late miscarriage, pre-term birth, premature rupture of membranes, low birth-weight and infection after delivery. It is also thought to increase the risk of contracting HIV.[11]

Cystitis (urinary tract infection)

The most common age to present with urinary tract infection (UTI) symptoms as an adult is the mid twenties. A total of 36% of women suffer a recurrence of symptoms within one year and 75% within two years. In 80% of cases the recurrence is due to a reinfection. A UTI is an extremely common reason for a visit to a general practitioner, accounting for between 1 and 6% of consultations.

Vaginal intercourse has an effect on susceptibility to UTIs, although the exact mechanism remains unknown. Episodes of cystitis are often associated with the onset of sexual intercourse and women having regular intercourse have three to four times as many episodes of infection per year compared to those not having intercourse.[12]

Signs and symptoms
A UTI may cause one or more of the following symptoms:

- a burning feeling in the urethra on urination; sometimes there can be blood in the urine or it may be cloudy
- needing to pass water very frequently, even when little urine is present
- a dragging ache in the lower back or abdomen.

UTIs can be caused by:

- bacteria – from the bowel
- friction – during sex
- 'irritable bladder' – a particularly sensitive bladder.

Diagnosis and treatment
There are over-the-counter treatments for UTIs. For milder cases there are also several home remedies that can alleviate the symptoms:

- drinking lots of water (or any other bland liquid) to flush out bacteria and dilute the urine so that it does not sting as much when urinating
- taking a teaspoon of bicarbonate of soda mixed with half a pint of water, or other bland liquid, every hour. This makes the urine less acidic and stops bacteria multiplying. It also eases the stinging sensation when passing urine
- taking painkillers
- some women find that drinking cranberry juice regularly can help clear up an attack.

If symptoms persist, the doctor will need a sample of urine to find out whether there is an infection and antibiotics are required.

How to avoid a UTI
- Always wipe your bottom from front to back.
- Drink plenty of bland fluids.
- Avoid perfumed products in the genital area.
- Wash and pass water before and after sex.

Hepatitis

Hepatitis is inflammation of the liver. This can be caused by alcohol and some drugs, but usually it is the result of a viral infection. There are several viruses that cause hepatitis. Both hepatitis B and C can persist in the body and may cause chronic liver damage. Each of these viruses acts differently; this section describes the most common forms of hepatitis that can be passed on through sexual intercourse.

Hepatitis A

It is difficult to ascertain the prevalence of hepatitis A within the population. Cases of hepatitis A infection may not be detected through GUM clinic attendances as such infections do not present. Sexual transmission is not the only route by which hepatitis A is passed on and its symptoms are general and not necessarily indicative of an STI, therefore clients are more likely to present to their GP.

Laboratory reports show that hepatitis A prevalence has greatly decreased over the last decade (*see* Table 7.2);[11] this is probably due to increased awareness and vaccination. Hepatitis A diagnosis is most common in the 15–34 age group, where it has actually increased over the past few years. This could be attributable to increased sexual activity, world travel and lack of awareness of risk. Diagnoses are

Table 7.2 Hepatitis A laboratory reports, England and Wales, by age group[11]

Age group (years)	1990	2000	2001	2002
Less than 1	9	2	1	2
1–4	272	29	19	26
5–14	2015	162	129	113
15–24	1670	242	195	458
25–34	1782	249	174	434
35–44	861	132	92	139
45–54	345	77	62	56
55–64	194	43	24	47
Greater than 65	132	70	73	65
Not known	265	42	20	12
TOTAL	**7545**	**1048**	**789**	**1352**

Table 7.3 Hepatitis A laboratory reports, England and Wales, by sex[11]

	1990	2000	2001	2002
Male	3990	632	494	908
Female	3457	396	279	428
Not known	98	20	16	16

greater in males than females (*see* Table 7.3),[11]probably due to a higher prevalence amongst men who have sex with men.

Signs and symptoms

People with hepatitis A may not have symptoms but can still be infectious. Symptoms may include:

- a short, flu-like illness
- fatigue
- nausea and vomiting
- diarrhoea
- loss of appetite
- weight loss
- jaundice
- itchy skin.

How it is passed on

- It is possible to become infected through eating or drinking contaminated food or water.
- The virus is found in faeces and can be passed on if even a tiny amount of virus comes into contact with a person's mouth. This means that the virus can also be passed on sexually. (Hand-washing after going to the toilet and before eating is important.)

Diagnosis and treatment

Hepatitis A is diagnosed by a blood test. There may be evidence of past infection which means there has been contact with hepatitis A but there were no obvious symptoms. This might provide protection from future infection with hepatitis A. Infection is usually mild but some people may need to be admitted to hospital.

A single injection of hepatitis A vaccine in the arm will give you protection for one year. A second booster injection at 6–12 months gives protection for up to ten years. Immunisation is recommended if you are travelling to parts of the world with high rates of hepatitis A. People who have been in recent contact with someone with hepatitis A may also be offered immunoglobulin to help try to prevent infection.

Hepatitis B

Laboratory reports show that hepatitis B figures have remained relatively constant over the last decade (*see* Table 7.4).[13] It is most common in those aged 25–34 years and prevalence is significantly higher amongst men (*see* Table 7.5);[13] this is probably due to increased sexual activity in this age group and men who have sex with men, respectively.

Signs and symptoms

People with hepatitis B may not have symptoms but can still be infectious. Symptoms may include:

- a short, flu-like illness
- fatigue

Table 7.4 Hepatitis B laboratory reports, England and Wales, by age group[13]

Age group (years)	1990	2000	2001	2002
Less than 1	3	1	1	1
1–4	3	2	0	1
5–9	3	4	0	2
10–14	8	2	1	5
15–24	184	175	144	193
25–34	187	242	176	264
35–44	109	115	126	181
45–54	53	68	64	89
55–64	26	35	22	48
Greater than 65	17	17	20	22
Not known	25	15	17	26
TOTAL	**618**	**676**	**571**	**832**

Table 7.5 Hepatitis B laboratory reports, England and Wales, by sex[13]

	1990	2000	2001	2002
Male	457	467	387	578
Female	159	191	169	238
Not known	2	18	15	16

- nausea and vomiting
- diarrhoea
- loss of appetite
- weight loss
- jaundice
- itchy skin.

How it is passed on
The hepatitis B virus is very common worldwide. It is very infectious and can be passed on in a number of ways:

- by unprotected penetrative sex
- by sharing needles or other drug-injecting equipment contaminated with blood
- by using equipment for tattooing, acupuncture or body-piercing contaminated with blood
- infected mothers may pass it on to their child during pregnancy or at birth
- through a blood transfusion in a country where blood is not tested (all blood for transfusion is tested in the UK).

Diagnosis and treatment
Hepatitis B is diagnosed by a blood test. There may be evidence of past infection that means there has been contact with hepatitis B but there were no obvious

symptoms. This might provide natural protection from future infection with hepatitis B. If a blood test indicates that a person is a hepatitis B carrier, this means that they can pass it to others. They are also at risk of chronic liver disease and may be referred to a specialist for further assessment. If diagnosed as having an active infection, they will be advised to have regular blood tests and physical check-ups. Many people do not require treatment as inflammation of the liver may not be severe. Treatment may be by interferon injections or antiviral tablets which can reduce hepatitis B damage.

Protection against hepatitis B is given by immunisation in injection form. Three injections of hepatitis B vaccine are given over a period of three to six months. A blood test is then taken to check there is an adequate level of protection. Immunisation lasts for at least five years. It is important that babies of hepatitis B-positive mothers are immunised at birth to prevent them from becoming infected.

Hepatitis C

Most hepatitis C infection is in the 25–34 and 35–44 age groups, with more reports in males than females (*see* Tables 7.5 and 7.6).[13] Risk factor information indicates the most common risk factor is injecting drug use (80%), followed by receipt of blood products and transfusions (10%). Multiple sexual partners, sexual

Table 7.6   Hepatitis C laboratory reports, England and Wales, by age group[13]

Age group (years)	1990	2000	2001	2002
Less than 1	0	2	9	3
1–4	1	8	8	25
5–14	9	13	15	23
15–24	9	686	551	686
25–34	67	1944	1652	2039
35–44	58	1386	1384	1734
45–54	20	722	718	832
55–64	25	155	175	208
Greater than 65	27	196	214	211
Not known	25	124	159	156
TOTAL	**241**	**5236**	**4885**	**5917**

Table 7.7   Hepatitis C laboratory reports, England and Wales, by sex[13]

	1990	2000	2001	2002
Male	160	3406	3260	4051
Female	74	1645	1470	1748
Not known	7	185	155	118

health clinic attendance and prostitution are also associated with an increased risk of hepatitis C infection.[14]

Signs and symptoms
People with hepatitis C may not have symptoms but can still be infectious. Symptoms may include:

• a flu-like illness
• fatigue
• nausea and vomiting
• diarrhoea
• weight loss
• jaundice in a small number of cases
• itchy skin.

How it is passed on
The hepatitis C virus can be spread in the following ways:

• by sharing needles or other drug-injecting equipment contaminated with blood
• by using equipment for tattooing, acupuncture or body-piercing contaminated with blood
• by unprotected penetrative sex
• infected mothers may pass it on to their child during pregnancy or at birth
• through a blood transfusion in a country where blood is not tested (all blood for transfusion is tested in the UK).

Diagnosis and treatment
Hepatitis C is diagnosed by a blood test. The first blood test will show whether an individual has ever been exposed to hepatitis C and a further blood test is necessary to establish whether they remain infected with the virus. After a number of years infection with hepatitis C can lead to the following conditions:

• chronic hepatitis
• liver cirrhosis
• liver cancer.

A few people experience recurrent attacks of flu-like illness and/or chronic fatigue. Those who have current infection should be referred to a specialist for further assessment; this will include liver function tests (a blood test) and possibly a biopsy (taking a small sample of liver tissue for examination). The results of these investigations will help the specialist decide whether treatment will be beneficial. The current medical treatment is the drug alpha interferon. It is not suitable for everybody but some patients can be successfully treated and it will clear the virus.

Infestations

Infestations occur where there is skin-to-skin contact, hence they are associated with sexual intercourse.

Pubic lice

The exact incidence of pubic lice is unknown, but it is common amongst young adults.[13]

Signs and symptoms
The most common symptom is itching in the infected areas. It may be possible to see droppings from the lice in underwear (black powder) and eggs on pubic or other hair; it is sometimes possible to see lice on the skin.

Transmission
Pubic lice are usually sexually transmitted but can occasionally be transferred by close physical contact or by sharing sheets or towels.

Diagnosis and treatment
The lice can be detected by physical examination and may be examined under a microscope. Special shampoo or lotion can easily stop the infestation. Any partners of the infected person should also be treated.

Scabies

Scabies has a cyclical rise in incidence roughly every 20 years in the UK. Reported cases have risen in the UK since 1991, often presenting as outbreaks in schools and residential or nursing homes. Scabies is more prevalent in urban than rural areas, and in winter than in summer. It is also more prevalent in children and young adults, but all ages can be affected.[15]

Signs and symptoms
The main symptom of scabies is an itchy rash on hands, wrists, elbows, underneath arms, abdomen, breasts, genitals or buttocks.

Transmission
Scabies is not necessarily sexually transmitted; any close physical contact can spread the infection.

Diagnosis and treatment
The rash can be seen on physical examination and may be examined under a microscope. Scabies is easily treated by special shampoo or lotion. Any partners of the infected person should also be treated.

HIV and AIDS

By the end of 2002 the estimated number of people living with HIV in the UK was estimated at 49 500, an increase of 20% compared with 2001. In 2002, 5700 new HIV cases were diagnosed. This was more than double the number diagnosed in 1998. The numbers of AIDS diagnoses and deaths in HIV-infected individuals declined after the introduction of effective therapies in the mid 1990s, and in more recent years have remained relatively constant.[16]

Sex between men and women overtook sex between men as the most common route of HIV transmission in 1999. The 3300 new HIV infections diagnosed in 2002 that were heterosexually acquired represent more than three times the number in 1996, when fewer than 900 such infections were diagnosed. Two-thirds of those diagnosed in 2002 were in women, and three-quarters of the total in both men and women (2500) were attributed to infection in Africa.[15]

What's the difference between HIV and AIDS?

HIV (human immunodeficiency virus) is the virus that causes AIDS (acquired immunodeficiency syndrome). AIDS is a serious condition in which the body's defences against some illnesses have broken down. This means that people with AIDS are vulnerable to many different diseases that a healthy person's body would normally deal with quite easily.

How long does it take for HIV to cause AIDS?

The length of time between being infected with HIV and being diagnosed with AIDS depends on many variables. Currently there are drugs that can be used to offset the development of AIDS from HIV.

How is a person infected?

HIV is passed on via the sexual fluids or blood of an infected person. This usually happens through sexual intercourse or by sharing needles. Mothers may pass HIV to a child at childbirth; it can also be passed through breast milk and a very small number of people become infected by having medical treatment using infected blood transfusions (all blood is screened for infection in the UK).

Oral sex carries some risk of infection. Infected fluid could get into the mouth where the virus enters into the blood via bleeding gums or sores. Infection from oral sex alone is very rare.

How is a person tested for HIV and AIDS?

HIV is detected via a blood test. It is advised to wait three months after the last risky sexual contact before having the test. This is because the virus is not detectable before this 'window period' has elapsed.

References

1   www.hpa.org.uk (2004)
2   Health Protection Agency (2002) New episodes of gonorrhoea by gender and age, 1995–2000. *Social Trends*. **32**.
3   Thivolet J (1980) Genital herpes. *Revue Française de Gynocologie et d'Obstetrique*. **75** (3): 79–81.
4   British National Association for Sexual Health and HIV: www.mssvd.org.uk (2004)

5   Petrin D, Delgarty K, Bhatt R *et al.* (1998) Clinical and microbiological aspects of *Trichomonas vaginalis. Clinical Medical Reviews.* **11** (2): 300–17.

6   Wolner-Hannsen P (1997) PID and obstetric infections. *Current Opinion in Infectious Diseases.* **10** (1): 50–4.

7   www.avert.org.stdstatisticuk.htm

8   Fieldhouse R (2001) The return of syphilis. *AIDS Treatment Update.* **103**: 2–5.

9   Kell P, McMarrow S and Smith A (2000) Management of syphilis in pregnancy. *CME Bulletin of Sexually Transmitted Infections and HIV.* **4** (1): 9–12.

10   Sanchez PJ (2002) Central nervous system infection in congenital syphilis. *New England Journal of Medicine.* **346** (23): 1792–8.

11   Health Protection Agency (2002) *CDR Weekly.* **12** (22): 8–10.

12   www.link.med.ed.ac.uk/RIDU/UTI2.htm

13   Health Protection Agency (2003) *Laboratory Reports to CDSC.* HPA, London.

14   Booth JCL, O'Grady J and Neuberger J (2001) *Clinical Guidance on the Management of Hepatitis C.* Compiled on behalf of the Royal College of Physicians of London and the British Society of Gastroenterology.

15   www.prodigy.nhs.uk (2004)

16   Health Protection Agency (2004) HIV and AIDS: diagnoses and deaths in HIV-infected individuals. *Social Trends.* **34**.

Resources
Information for young people

- www.playingsafely.co.uk
  NHS website on sexual health for young people; it includes good interactive games highlighting the 'STI lottery' of unprotected sexual intercourse.

- www.avert.org
  Information for young people about HIV infection and AIDS, sex, puberty, sexuality, contraception and condoms. Includes personal stories, articles and resources such as quizzes, statistics, frequently asked questions (FAQs) and printable booklets.

- www.lovelife.uk.com
  Features information and advice on STIs and how to avoid them, where to go for a check-up and emergency help, and how to use condoms correctly.

- www.nhsdirect.nhs.uk/SelfHelp/info/advice/stis.stm
  Straightforward but brief outline of STIs and their treatments. Part of the NHS Direct website.

Advice for young people

- *Brook*
  Helpline: 0800 0185 023 (Mondays to Thursdays, 9am–5pm; Fridays, 9am–4pm)
  Website: www.brook.org.uk

Provides free and confidential contraceptive advice for anyone under 25, and emergency contraception, pregnancy testing and counselling on any sex and relationship problem. 24-hour recorded messages on pregnancy, contraception, abortion and STIs: 020 7617 8000.

- *Association for Genito-Urinary Medicine (AGUM)*
  www.agum.org.uk/directory.htm
  Online directory of GUM (sexual health) clinics for the UK and Republic of Ireland.

- *Society of Health Advisers in Sexually Transmitted Diseases*
  www.shastd.org.uk
  Contains answers to FAQs about STIs, information about infections and treatments, a discussion forum and details of GUM clinics around the UK.

Literature

- *Family Planning Association (fpa)*
  2–12 Pentonville Road, London N1 9FP
  Leaflets on STIs are also available on their website: www.fpa.org.uk

- Mason M-C (2002) *Sexually Transmitted Infections*. Sheldon Press, London. This guide to sexual health discusses most STIs and explains their diagnosis, symptoms, treatment and prevention.

- *HIV and AIDS: information for young people*
  Booklet downloadable from www.avert.org/ypbooks.htm

Information for professionals

- www.prodigy.nhs.uk
  Prodigy is a broad concept to support general practice in developing the quality of clinical practice. It uses computers to support decision making within the consultation, to enable easy access to knowledge in an educational context and to support reflection through personal and practice benchmarking (improving ourselves by learning from others) using computer queries.

- www.hpa.org.uk
  The Health Protection Agency (HPA) is a national organisation for England and Wales, established on 1 April 2003. It is dedicated to protecting people's health and reducing the impact of infectious diseases, chemical hazards, poisons and radiation hazards. It brings together the expertise of health and scientific professionals working in public health, communicable disease, emergency planning, infection control and poisons, chemical, and radiation hazards.

- The Brook (www.brook.org.uk) and AVERT (www.avert.org) websites also have factual information and research for professionals.

CHAPTER 8

Marginalised groups

This chapter focuses on the sexual health issues of specific marginalised groups within society. These groups have been identified as excluded by the Social Exclusion Unit in the Teenage Pregnancy Strategy and include:[1] looked-after children, some ethnic groups, young people who are at greater risk of becoming involved in or are already involved in prostitution, young men, young people with disabilities and lesbian, gay, bisexual and transgender young people.

Ethnic groups

Statistics

One in every 11 15–19 year-olds in Great Britain is from a minority ethnic group. Half live in London, a quarter in the West Midlands, West Yorkshire and Greater Manchester and the rest throughout the country.[2]

Teenage motherhood and prevalence of STIs are generally more common amongst ethnic groups. Statistics between different ethnic groups vary widely and the reasons underlying this are a complex mixture of cultural, behavioural, social and economic factors.

Teenage motherhood

People from ethnic groups are more likely to live in deprived areas and poverty. Teenage motherhood is more common in black Caribbean, Pakistani and Bang-ladeshi groups than in white ethnic groups.[2] How poverty can influence teenage pregnancy rates has been discussed in Chapter 4. Having a baby is not perceived as interfering with life goals in lower social classes and therefore young women tend to become mothers sooner than their peers in higher social classes. Abortion rates amongst teenagers illustrate this: in deprived areas 25–30% of pregnancies are terminated whereas the figure is 60% in affluent areas.[3] Teen mothers are less likely to achieve the same levels of education and employment as their childless peers and often the poverty cycle is perpetuated.

However, it is important to realise that poverty is only one of a number of factors influencing teen pregnancy rates in ethnic groups. Religious and cultural beliefs and practices often support teenage motherhood within marriage. Evidence suggests that for young people from Afro-Caribbean, Bangladeshi, Pakistani Muslim and traveller communities there is a high incidence of early pregnancy, mostly within marriage. In Afro-Caribbean communities there are strong pro-fertility beliefs, where large families are seen as a source of economic asset and strength. Within Asian families, teenage marriage followed by pregnancy is the norm. Delaying conception, having smaller families and motherhood out of marriage can lead to conflict with cultural and religious traditions.[4]

Sexually transmitted infections

Teenagers from black Caribbean backgrounds are at highest risk of gonorrhoea and chlamydia per head of population. Other STI distribution does not vary significantly by ethnic group. HIV/AIDs is uncommon amongst teenagers, though a disproportionate number of 15–19 year-olds from black African backgrounds were being treated for HIV in 2000: 42 out of a total of 104. This does not necessarily mean that these groups are more promiscuous. Sexual partners tend to come from within the same ethnic group; therefore an infection can circulate at high levels within one group and be rare in another, despite similar sexual behaviour levels.[2]

Attitudes within community groups

A strong and positive community identity gives a sense of place and self-esteem to individual members. Faith identities can help to build self-esteem and reduce pressure from wider cultural influences, such as the media and peers, to engage in unsafe sexual activities. If an individual has high self-esteem they are more likely to put positive sexual health messages into practice. Conversely, if a cultural group has experienced historical and current rejection, it can have a negative impact on self-perception and increase risk-taking behaviours.

Cultural practices are often linked to religious beliefs. Religion plays a strong role in influencing attitudes towards behaviours such as premarital sex or same-sex intercourse. Young people brought up in strict, religiously observant households tend to hold less permissive attitudes towards sexual behaviour. Whilst this may influence young people to delay sexual intercourse or reserve it for marriage, it can also lead to feelings of guilt if they do enter a sexual relationship before marriage and fear of accessing services in case family members find out. In an extended family personal privacy may be seen as unnecessary, personal information is public knowledge and professional confidentiality may be viewed with suspicion. Behaviour that is in breach of cultural and/or religious norms may bring shame on a family. Any resultant delay in accessing services can put young people from these groups at risk of untreated sexual infections or single parenthood.

Policy and action

The Teenage Pregnancy Strategy[1] aims to improve information about ethnic variation in teenage conceptions and address the needs of minority ethnic communities in local plans. The National Strategy for Sexual Health and HIV proposes strategies to address the prevention needs of black and minority ethnic groups.[5]

There are many religious groups represented in the UK and specific issues are examined in the Government document *Diverse Communities: identity and teenage pregnancy*,[4] which is a resource for practitioners.

For practitioners, a community profile will highlight the ethnic communities represented locally. Statistics about health, poverty and social exclusion should be researched for each community as they will vary for different subgroups.

The benefits of delaying pregnancy for health, educational or socio-economic reasons need to be openly explained during consultation with community organisations as part of an overall health agenda. It is vital to consult with local organisations to dispel their fears over their young people being corrupted. Consulting with young people from ethnic groups and religious communities will ensure that services meet their specific needs.

Research carried out for the *Diverse Communities* resource showed that young people from these groups feel that:[4]

- their values are ignored and should be included in sex and relationships education (SRE)
- they are not given access to information about sexual health
- they are not always certain that confidentiality will be maintained
- they would like information and support from professionals that acknowledges their cultural and religious upbringing.

SRE in schools and youth groups should be inclusive of different faiths and cultures. Consultation with parents and young people will ensure that practice is not based on stereotypes and false assumptions.

Work with ethnic groups should focus on empowerment: developing positive ethnic/cultural identities which leads to increased self-esteem and gives young people the confidence to have control over what happens in their lives.

Young men
Excluded from services

Young men/fathers tend to be left out of service provision as services generally focus on contraceptive advice; the majority of methods are for women so young men see these services as irrelevant for them. As a result they are not actively encouraged to be involved in decisions regarding fertility control and they may withdraw from taking responsibility for contraceptive and sexual health issues within a relationship.

Research shows that when young men become fathers they would like to be more involved in the decision-making process around pregnancy and care of their children.[6] Some young men may have very strong views about pregnancy. Yet when a partner becomes pregnant there is very little support available for young men to help deal with these issues. Advisory services should work to include young fathers in the decision-making process as, even if they don't get their preferred choice, they will be emotionally better off. Being connected to the consequences of unprotected sex means they are likely to take more responsibility in future relationships.

Research also shows that young fathers often want to stay in touch with their children and play a part in their upbringing. More often than not the relationship has broken down and they are denied access.[6] Fatherhood is confusing, and information and support are hard to find with few established networks for men or fathering.

The National Children's Bureau conducted a study on pregnancy and parenthood with young men and women. The study showed that girls had a poor opinion of young men's attitudes towards fatherhood. Fewer than a quarter thought that young men took their responsibilities seriously. Conversely, almost two-thirds of the boys felt they did take responsibility within a relationship. While some young mothers were ambivalent about the role they wished the baby's father to play in their lives, many were inclined to reject the father, preferring to struggle alone rather than accept what they viewed as inadequate offers of help from an unreliable partner. The study also showed that there is little evidence of young mothers being actively encouraged to maintain a relationship with the baby's father. It is rare to find supported accommodation where fathers can be involved with their partner and child, and this only serves to drive fathers further out of the picture.[7]

Work with young men

Work with young men and young fathers should be an intrinsic part of work around teenage pregnancy and parenthood and not an additional extra. To be relevant and appealing to young men, projects need to be broader than just giving information on contraception. They need to address personal issues and work with emotional and lifestyle factors. For many young men, lifestyle, growing up, self-image and self-esteem are the important issues in their lives. They may engage in high risk-taking behaviour, have low emotional literacy, low motivation, low levels of educational attainment, suffer from depression and place an emphasis on material wealth. Projects need to deal with these issues alongside those such as parenting.

Any service set up for young men should be based on an assessment of their needs, and for it to be effective, the young men themselves should be involved in its development. To attract and engage young men, outreach work needs to be creative and fun, e.g. through music, art and sport. These can be used to promote important sexual health messages. As the trust of the young men is built up they

---

Box 8.1   The Young African-Caribbean Men's Sexual Health Project[1]

Role Model sessions have been used within a local school as part of a mentoring project. A group of African-Caribbean young men invite professionals to visit the group and talk about how they got into their profession. The group also holds sessions (amongst other subjects) on sexual health. The young people set the curriculum for the group and a health promotion specialist facilitates the sessions. The project has begun to identify areas of concern to do with attitudes to women and sexual relationships.

Several research sessions have been held with young African-Caribbean people that focused on relationship issues between men and women. The purpose of these experimental sessions was to identify young people's views and the issues that are important to them. It is hoped that this will be useful in informing the development of future work. They used a daytime TV talkshow format as this is familiar to the group.

may ask questions and stay to talk. For example, in Camden and Islington in London, the Young African-Caribbean Men's Sexual Health Project has a range of innovative and culturally appropriate initiatives to raise awareness on various health and social issues. A couple of examples are given in Box 8.1.

It is important that staff working with young men are empathetic and tolerant. Young men may behave in ways that staff find uncomfortable, but this has to be worked with if trust and rapport are to develop. Young men respond to staff who respect confidentiality, understand youth culture and are non-judgemental.[8]

Group work can be combined with one-to-one support. Young men can maintain their image in the group and deal with sensitive issues in one-to-one sessions. Group work can be used to discuss embarrassing and sensitive issues with their peers. Both approaches can help develop their emotional literacy.

Young people with disabilities

Disabled children represent approximately 3% of the child population.[9] They are less likely to receive both formal and informal sex education and can be ill-equipped to deal with emerging emotions and developing relationships.

If we are to treat people with disabilities as equal members of society, we must not deny them the opportunity to understand their sexuality in terms of their body and their emotions. All children have a legal right to education and support that will prepare them for the responsibilities and experiences of adult life. In addition, disabled children are more likely to suffer sexual abuse than their non-disabled peers; it is vital that they receive support to develop an awareness of physical boundaries. (*See* Chapter 4 for information regarding abuse and child protection.)

Sex and relationships education

Sex and relationships education (SRE) is an important part of the curriculum for all young people. Disabled young people are less likely to receive sex education in school and at home, and their experiences are often excluded or misrepresented in the media, where other children pick up information. This can leave disabled young people ill-equipped to develop fulfilling sexual relationships and lead to loneliness and isolation.[10]

A lack of knowledge around emotional and physical boundaries and sexual health may mean that young people with disabilities cannot make informed decisions within relationships and may not be aware when these boundaries are being abused. Sex education can be a form of protection from abuse.

Under the provisions of the Special Educational Needs and Disability Act,[11] schools are required to ensure that the curriculum (including PSHE and SRE) meets the needs of disabled students. SRE classes should involve tasks that everyone can achieve at their own level. Young people with learning disabilities may need additional learning opportunities and reinforcement. SRE resources should be inclusive and provide positive images of disabled young people.

Often it is the attitudes of service providers and families that present obstacles to people with disabilities leading sexual lives or developing relationships. Non-disabled people may have difficulty accepting that disabled people can have fulfilling sex lives. Parents of disabled children may be reticent for their children to explore sexual relationships due to fears over them being abused or find it difficult to accept they are developing into an adult. For parents who want to provide sex education for their children, many are unsure how to do it.

Higher risk of abuse

Young people with disabilities are at a higher risk of abuse.[12] Systematic data collection and research in the UK relating to child protection or abuse of disabled children are lacking; however, an American study of over 40 000 children found that disabled children were 3.4 times more likely to be abused and, more specifically, 3.1 times more likely to be sexually abused than their non-disabled peers.[13]

Furthermore, disabled children in residential accommodation are extremely vulnerable to abuse of all kinds, including abuse from peers.[14] Recent research indicates that men with learning disabilities make up the biggest single group of known perpetrators of sexual abuse against other people with learning disabilities.[15]

The following are factors that contribute to young people with disabilities being more vulnerable to sexual abuse:

- Compliance and passivity are qualities that are often fostered and rewarded in disabled children. Together with possible poor self-image and low self-esteem, it can be difficult for them to resist abuse.
- The idea of private parts has limited meaning for children who require help with basic toileting and dressing functions.
- Young disabled people often receive intimate personal care, possibly from a number of carers. This may increase the risk of exposure to abusive behaviour.
- Due to personal care being carried out by someone else, they can lack awareness of the physical boundaries that able-bodied children learn.
- Isolation and inexperience arising from reduced social experiences through disability may mean that they are unaware of appropriate behaviour in social interaction.
- A specific disability may mean they may have an impaired capacity to resist or avoid abuse.

The disability itself, such as an inability to speak or to understand what is happening, can make it difficult for young people with a disability to disclose what is happening to a trusted person. Even if physically and mentally able, mobility problems or reduced independence means young people with disabilities are likely to have less social contacts and may simply not know who to tell. In addition, as discussed earlier, young people with disabilities are less likely to receive sex education than their mainstream counterparts and may not know that they are being abused.

Outreach

There should be consultation with young people with disabilities in matters related to their care. Only then will provision tackle issues that are relevant to them. It is important to ensure that there are effective networks and support

Box 8.2   The Limelight Project[16]

The Limelight Project is for disabled people over the age of 18. Peer educators work alongside other disabled people as their ally in ways that are empowering, enabling and supportive. The project aims to challenge some of the myths, prejudices, misconceptions and taboos associated with sexuality and disability.

Based at the Family Planning Association in Belfast, Northern Ireland, its aim is to train approximately 20 disabled people, to an accredited level, to be peer educators on issues concerning sexuality and disability.

These peer educators facilitate workshops for community groups on issues concerning disability, sexuality and relationships; and provide input into training for professionals working in the area of sexuality and relationships.

---

systems in place. Due to a reduced ability to freely access community provision, services need to be innovative to be effective. One good example is the Limelight Project in Belfast, where peer educators discuss sex and relationship issues with young disabled people and provide positive role models (*see* Box 8.2).[16]

SRE workshops can be carried out in schools and youth groups. Storytelling and use of scenarios are good ways of exploring relationships. This is useful for young people who have reduced opportunities to meet people and form relationships and fewer opportunities to learn and practise relevant skills.

Props are essential for illustrating sexual health messages. These should be tailored to the group, e.g. large print for the visually impaired, anatomically correct models for those with learning disabilities, etc.

Working with parents is also important to reduce any fears and worries they may have regarding their disabled child's emerging sexuality. As well as drawing support from other parents, group facilitators can direct parents to useful resources for discussing issues around sexual health and development at home (see list at the end of the chapter for suggested resources).

Finally, it is important to have a clear policy on confidentiality to help to develop young people's trust. The lives of disabled children and young people are often so open to public scrutiny that they may feel that everything they do or say will be reported. A clear confidentiality policy that is made explicit will reassure them to the contrary. Chapter 10 looks at outreach work with young people in more detail.

Lesbian, gay, bisexual and transgender young people

Lesbian, gay, bisexual and transgender (LGBT) young people often feel isolated within a society that has mixed feelings about sexuality that is not heterosexual. Young people often experience bullying from peers, fear over non-acceptance by family and friends, and difficulty developing relationships for fear of reactions around them.

Emerging sexuality

Sexuality is fluid. Many people have feelings towards other people of the same sex at some point in their lives. Some people who are attracted to people of the same sex are homosexual and go on to have sexual relationships with people of the same sex. Other people who have homosexual feelings find that these change over time and they become attracted to people of the opposite sex. Other people are attracted to both men and women and have relationships with both. Some people are not attracted to anyone. There is evidence that for some people homosexual experiences may well be part of a transitional or experimental phase in their youth. For many people these feelings can be very intense and alienating. It is vital to provide a nurturing support system so that young people experiencing these feelings can explore their sexuality safely.

Societal attitude

Varying sexual orientations are increasingly accepted in society. Research carried out in 1996 by Stonewall showed that people who are homosexual had experienced extreme homophobia as young people; 90% of the respondents had been called names and nearly 50% had been violently attacked.[17]

Statistics

Between 1989 and 1990, a National Survey of Sexual Attitudes and Lifestyles (NATSAL) of nearly 19 000 people was undertaken in Britain. The survey examined a cross-section of people throughout the country, looking at their sexual

Table 8.1 National Survey of Sexual Attitudes and Lifestyles by sex[18,19]

	Men NATSAL I % 1990	Men NATSAL II % 2000	Women NATSAL I % 1990	Women NATSAL II % 2000
Ever had a sexual experience, not necessarily including genital contact, with a partner of the same sex?	5.3	8.4	2.8	9.7
Ever had sex with a same-sex partner, including genital contact?	3.7	6.3	1.9	5.7
Have you had a same-sex partner in the last five years?	1.4	2.6	0.6	2.6

Table 8.2   National Survey of Sexual Attitudes and Lifestyles by sex and age group[18,19]

	NATSAL I % 1990	NATSAL II % 2000 16–17 yrs	18–19 yrs	20–24 yrs	*Average 16–24 yrs*
		Men			
Ever had a sexual experience with a same-sex partner?	4.3	1.2	5.6	6.3	**4.3**
Ever had sexual intercourse/ genital contact with a same-sex partner?	2.4	1.2	2.3	4.2	**2.6**
		Women			
Ever had a sexual experience with a same-sex partner?	3.0	5.1	9.7	12.6	**9.1**
Ever had sexual intercourse/ genital contact with a same-sex partner?	1.4	2.5	4.6	6.5	**4.5**

attitudes and behaviour, including people's same-sex sexual experiences. It was repeated in 1999–2001. The results of the study provide an interesting comparison of how same-sex sexual behaviour is changing in Britain (*see* Table 8.1).[18,19]

The study shows either that same-sex sexual behaviour is on the increase or that people are more willing to report it. In 2000, 91.9% of men and 88.3% of women said they had only ever had sexual attraction towards the opposite sex, therefore it can be assumed that 8.1% of men and 11.7% of women have felt a sexual attraction towards the same sex at least once in their lives. The study also looked at men's and women's experiences by age group (*see* Table 8.2).[18,19] The difference between 1990 and 2000 is most apparent in young women, where same-sex sexual experience rose from 3% in 1990 to 9.1% in 2000. For men, the data show that same-sex sexual experience increases more rapidly over the age of 18 years.

Bullying

Young men and women who do not act in line with gender stereotypes may be subjected to bullying by their peers. Boys appear to be more prejudiced than girls towards homosexual people.[20] This could be because the boundaries of boys' gender roles tend to be much more rigid than they are for girls. Boys have a limited number of ways to express their emotions that are acceptable to their peer group. This often means that any emotional expression between boys may be seen as homosexual interest by their peers. In contrast, between girls, close friendships (which often involve embracing, touching, and sharing thoughts and feelings) are more legitimate and less likely to be seen by their peers as an indication of homosexuality.

The word 'gay' is often used by young people as an insult. Communication is a complex affair in which not only the words used matter, but also who is saying them, about whom and in what context. A person called 'gay' by bullies in school might find it abusive because of the way it is said, but the same person might happily call themselves 'gay' when they are with friends.

The derogatory use of words associated with homosexuality is one way in which young people learn it is 'undesirable' to be homosexual. This can silence young people who are experiencing homosexual feelings. In order to protect themselves, young gay men often pretend to be heterosexual and sometimes join in homophobic taunts. Homosexual young people can be kept separate from each other because of the implications of being seen together by their peers. Patterns set down in adolescence can affect individuals for many years to come, often into their adult lives.

Coming out

LGBT young people face the difficulty of telling their parents and friends about their sexual orientation and helping them adjust to the news. Ineffective communication, poor self-esteem, and unresolved grief and anger often complicate the issue.

For ethnic minority LGBT young people, the 'coming out' process presents challenges in their identity formation processes and in their loyalties to one community over another. For example, they need to live within three rigidly defined and strongly independent communities: the gay and lesbian community, the ethnic community and society at large. It requires a constant effort to maintain themselves in different worlds, each of which fails to support significant aspects of their life.

Supporting young people who are exploring their sexuality

LGBT young people need help and support to understand the feelings they may be experiencing. Many LGBT adults say that they began to identify themselves as 'different' in their secondary school years. In this period, the absence of support, understanding or information is sometimes a source of distress in itself and often magnifies anxiety:

> I was waiting and expecting to hear something about homosexuality, safe sex and different things in sex education. Maybe some information that could help me. But I got nothing.[21]

SRE work in schools and outreach work in youth organisations should include positive information about same-sex relationships. Homophobic language and bullying should be challenged by adults. Professionals working with young people should be able to direct them to organisations that can support their emerging sexuality.

Looked-after children/children in residential care

Many young people who are in the care system have not had positive role models from which they can learn to form their own healthy, fulfilling relationships. Often young people in the care system are looking for love or someone to love and do this through sexual relationships. Frequent moves and a higher incidence of truancy can mean that vital sex education in school is missed. These factors lead to a disproportionately high number of young women leaving care who are pregnant, are already parents, or who become parents soon after.

Local authorities are duty bound under the terms of the Children Act 1989 to provide young people in their care with the knowledge and skills they require for positive sexual relationships.[22]

Statistics

At any one time around 60 000 children are in care. Two-thirds live in foster care and one-tenth in children's homes.[23]

Children in care suffer a greater incidence of the factors that have been identified by the Social Exclusion Unit as increasing the risk of becoming teenage parents: living in poverty; having been in care or fostered; experiencing low educational achievements; truancy or social exclusion; not being involved in education, training or work post-16; being sexually abused; experiencing mental health problems; being in trouble with the police; belonging to an ethnic minority.[1]

Children in care and care leavers are almost 2.5 times more likely to become teenage parents than those brought up by both natural parents.[24] Further surveys have shown that one quarter of care leavers have had a child by the age of 16,[25] and almost half of the young women who leave care are mothers within 18–24 months.[26]

Disabled children are often over-represented in the population of looked-after children: the annual statistics for children who were looked after in England in 2000 show that 9% were disabled. Disabled children are also more likely to be in residential care than non-disabled children.[27] As described in the section on children with disabilities, they are also highly represented in abuse statistics.

Forming positive relationships

A study carried out by the National Children's Bureau into the views and experiences of young people in care on pregnancy and parenthood showed that both boys and girls in care aspire to marriage and parenthood at an early age. Being in a steady relationship before the age of 20 was of major importance for all young people both in care and not in care, but significantly more of the looked-after sample also wanted to be married or cohabiting and have a child by then. The difference between the boys' responses was especially marked: 80% of them wanted to be married or cohabiting and 55% wanted at least one child, as opposed to 42% and 30% respectively in the comparator sample. As for pregnancy, 79% of the teenagers in public care compared with 52% living with their families said teenage pregnancies happen because teenagers want someone to love.[25]

Many looked-after young people have not experienced positive relationships with adults and have not had the opportunity to learn about trust and respect. Feeling unloved and uncared for, they are more likely to enter into a sexual relationship without consideration of either the suitability of the partner or the implications of their actions. Unless they receive affection and learn to understand the nature of love and respect which is not contingent upon sex, they are likely to continue in their search for love through sexual relationships and parenthood.

Abuse

Looked-after young people in residential care are more vulnerable to abuse than those who live in families, and under-reporting of institutional abuse is common.[28] Two separate studies have shown that sexual abuse made up 17%[29] and 24%[30] of the types of abuse children in residential facilities reported. Young people in residential care are more at risk of physical and sexual assault from their peers than from staff. One study found that 13% of children had been taken advantage of sexually by a peer whilst in care.[31]

Evidence from UK institutional abuse inquiry reports shows that either many of the children who had been abused had not reported the abuse, or their allegations had not been forwarded to the appropriate authorities.[32] These inquiries have noted that young people's complaints about abuse were frequently ignored or discounted because of negative assumptions that were made about the character, behaviour and truthfulness of young people placed in residential care.

Children in care may not report abuse as they can feel powerless to influence what happens to them, embarrassed, or that they may not be believed. In addition, the secretive nature of sexual abuse means there may be fewer opportunities for external individuals to witness and report the incident.

For professionals working with young people, it is essential to be aware that young people in residential care are at higher risk of sexual abuse and to take very seriously any indication or allegation of abuse.

Sex and relationships education

Young people in public care, especially those in residential care, frequently have poor rates of school attendance. They can miss long periods of schooling due to changes in schools, not having a school place, being excluded or not attending regularly. Consequently, as well as adversely affecting their overall educational achievement, they are likely to miss out on sex and relationships education. This is not routinely provided by carers or social workers who are typically untrained in this area and unsure of their responsibilities.

A National Children's Bureau study showed that looked-after girls were far less likely than those in a comparative sample to have been given information on some crucial topics such as contraception (including emergency contraception), pregnancy and pressure to have sex. Looked-after boys reported having received less information than their comparator sample peers about pressure to have sex, sexual feelings, sexual relationships and accessing local health services.[7]

For the young women who had early pregnancies, the vast majority reported that they did not receive unbiased information from those involved in their care about their options, or counselling to aid their decision making. Unsupported and unsure what to do, the young women typically did nothing.[7]

Under the terms of the Children Act 1989, local authorities have a duty to provide the sex education of the children and young people they look after. They are responsible for preparing young people for adulthood as they leave care, including those young people who leave care as parents.[22]

Action

One of the objectives of Quality Protects, the Government's initiative to improve local authority services for children, is to ensure that the number of pregnancies to girls under 16 in public care does not differ from that of the general population.[33]

Local authorities should have policies and guidelines on SRE for young people in public care. Input is vital if the young people are to receive the information necessary for forming positive, healthy relationships. Professionals working with children in care on SRE should be supported and trained in its delivery.

Young people in care should be consulted to find out the areas in which they lack SRE knowledge and also what are the contributing factors to their not receiving this input. Resultant projects will then be more effective and tailored to their needs. Projects may include work with foster carers and adoptive parents, outreach work in residential homes and one-to-one work.

Children involved in or at risk of becoming involved in prostitution

It is difficult to keep track of the numbers of children involved as the nature of child prostitution is secretive and based on fear.

Who is at risk?

Certain groups of young people are particularly vulnerable to becoming involved in child prostitution; for example, those who have become distanced from family and friends through various circumstances such as abuse in the family, being in care, truancy or exclusion from school. Adults who are looking to take advantage of children sexually are skilled at identifying disaffected, unhappy and vulnerable young people.

A study by leading children's charities and funded by the Home Office called 'More Than One Chance' interviewed 41 people aged between 14 and 38 with experience of prostitution. The interviews revealed that:[34]

- all of those interviewed had made more than one attempt to leave prostitution but felt there was not enough support to do so
- those interviewed feared violence from pimps far more than the violence they might suffer after getting into a car with a stranger
- the average age of their first experience of prostitution was 16 (some of those interviewed had been involved in prostitution since the age of 11)
- 77% of those interviewed had run away from home at least once and 83% had taken or were addicted to drugs before becoming involved in prostitution
- 75% of those interviewed had truanted from school
- everyone interviewed had suffered various forms of physical or sexual abuse at home
- the majority of interviewees felt they had little choice or control over their lives.

> One rent boy stated he had started selling sex at nine years old. The man who abused him gave him a bag of five pence pieces. By the age of 13 he was being shared around between a group of men.
>
> Another girl described the dangers of living on the streets. She was just 12 when she started running away from home. She said: 'A man approached me one time … I didn't want to do him and the geezer had me up by the throat, threatening to kill me. I was actually really scared, I didn't know whether he was going to knock me out or do what. They could just stab you, they could take you down an alley, they could rape you, then kill you. They could do anything.'[35]

The law and prosecution

Recently the law has shifted its focus from prosecuting child prostitutes to penalising those who are abusing the children either as coercionists or clients. This change has taken place through pressure from non-governmental organisations. Barnardo's produced a report in 1998 entitled 'Whose Daughter Next? Children Abused Through Prostitution', which was part of a campaign to raise awareness of the plight faced by children abused through prostitution. The report called for adults who abuse and exploit children for sex, power or money to be prosecuted in a way that reflects the seriousness of the crime.[36] As a result the Government now recognises that men who buy and sell sex from children should be called to account for breaking the law, while children abused in this way should be treated as children in need. Prostitution is not illegal. However, buying or selling sexual services on a street or in a public place is.

Pattern of abuse

A child may be physically and emotionally dependent on the coercionist despite the violence endured. Although the young person may claim to be acting voluntarily, this is not voluntary or consenting behaviour. The 'More Than One Chance' study showed that the controlling influence exerted by pimps is a major factor in preventing young people from leaving prostitution.[34]

During the course of its work with young women, Barnados has recognised a pattern of control and abuse in prostitution:[36]

- *ensnaring*, where a young man between 18 and 25 meets a girl, usually between 12 and 14, and impresses her with his maturity, money and good looks. They begin a sexual relationship and she falls in love
- *creating dependency*, where he becomes very possessive and destroys her ties to friends and family
- *taking control*, where he begins to control all aspects of her life and becomes violent
- *total dominance*, where she agrees to have sex with someone else, often one of his 'friends', without realising that money has changed hands.

Identifying children involved in prostitution

It may not always be obvious when a young person is involved in prostitution. Any concerns or uneasiness about an observed or reported relationship can be discussed with the child protection nurse specialist or doctor or the duty social worker.

Some examples could include:[37]

- a parent or carer may become aware of and concerned about a child's relationship with an older person
- staff working in a residential setting may become aware a child is being picked up by an unauthorised older person
- police may become aware of children involved in or at risk of entering into prostitution during investigation of drug offences, search warrants, etc.
- teachers will be aware of children who are not receiving affection and appropriate care within their families. This in turn isolates them from their peers and can lead to truancy and vulnerability to prostitution
- health professionals may be alerted when a young person seeks contraceptive and sexual health advice and treatment or requests termination of a pregnancy.

Looked-after children

Looked-after children who run away are particularly at risk of sexual exploitation. 'Missing From Care 1998', a report from a joint local government association and Association of Chief Police Officers working party, sets out recommended procedures and practices in caring for missing children and provides a basis on which such protocols may be developed.[38]

Safeguarding children involved in prostitution

The Government has guidelines to support agencies in identifying and dealing effectively with young people who are at risk of entering into or already involved in prostitution. The document, entitled 'Safeguarding Children Involved in Prostitution',[37] is to be used in conjunction with *Working Together to Safeguard Children*.[39] The main points of the document are that young people involved in prostitution should be treated as the victims of abuse and they are likely to require the provision of welfare services and protection under the Children Act 1989.

The document promotes an inter-agency approach whose aim is to safeguard and promote young people's welfare. A successful exit strategy from prostitution for a child is not simple and requires an inter-agency approach over a sustained period of time. It also encourages the investigation and prosecution of criminal activities by those who coerce children into, and abuse them through, prostitution.

The identification of a child involved in or at risk of being drawn into prostitution should always trigger local Area Child Protection Committee (ACPC) procedures to ensure the child's safety and welfare, and to enable the police to gather evidence about abusers and coercionists. (More details regarding this process are given in Chapter 3.)

The ACPC is a resource and source of expertise for those who have concerns that a child may be at risk of being drawn into, or is being abused through, prostitution. It will have a local protocol outlining how to respond to concerns. The ACPC can also provide training to raise awareness of issues pertaining to child prostitution.

References

1 Social Exclusion Unit (1999) *Teenage Pregnancy Strategy*. HMSO, London.
2 Low N (2001) *Sexual Health and Young People from Black and Minority Ethnic Groups*. University of Bristol, Bristol.
3 Brook (2003) *Teenage Conceptions: statistics and trends*. www.brook.org.uk/content/fact2_TeenageConceptions.pdf
4 Teenage Pregnancy Unit (2002) *Diverse Communities: identity and teenage pregnancy*. HMSO, London.
5 Department of Health (2001) *Sexual Health and HIV Strategy*. HMSO, London.
6 www.youngfathers.org.uk
7 Corlyon J and McGuire C (1999) *Pregnancy and Parenthood: the views and experiences of young people in public care*. National Children's Bureau, London.
8 Pearson S (2003) Men's use of sexual health services. *Journal of Family Planning and Reproductive Health Care*. **29** (4): 190–4.
9 Quality Protects (2000) *Disabled Children: numbers and categories and families*. HMSO, London.
10 Stewart D and Ray C (2001) *Ensuring Entitlement: sex and relationships education for disabled children*. Sex Education Forum, National Children's Bureau, London.
11 Department of Health (2001) *Special Educational Needs and the Disability Act*. HMSO, London.
12 McCarthy M (2000) Consent, abuse and choices: women with learning disabilities and sexuality. In: Traustadottir R and Johnson K (eds) (2000) *Women with Intellectual Disabilities: finding a place in the world*. Jessica Kingsley Publishers, London.

13   Sullivan PM and Knutson JF (2000) Maltreatment and disabilities: a population-based epidemiological study. *Child Abuse and Neglect.* **249** (10): 1257–73.

14   Department of Health (1997) *People Like Us: the report of the review of the safeguards for children living away from home.* HMSO, London.

15   McCarthy M and Thompson D (1992) *Sex and the 3 Rs: rights, responsibilities and risks. A sex education package for working with people with learning difficulties.* Pavilion Publishing, Brighton.

16   Family Planning Association (1999) *Executive Summary of the Evaluation Report.* FPA, London.

17   National Advisory Group (1999) *Breaking the Chain of Hate: a national survey examining levels of homophobic crime and community confidence towards the police service.* HMSO, London.

18   Wellings K, Field J and Johnson AM (1994) *National Survey of Sexual Attitudes and Lifestyles* I. National Centre for Social Research, London.

19   Erens B, McManus S, Prescott A *et al.* (2003) *National Survey of Sexual Attitudes and Lifestyles II: reference tables and summary report.* National Centre for Social Research, London.

20   Forrest S, Biddle G and Clift S (2003) *Talking About Homosexuality in the Secondary School.* AVERT. www.avert.org/ypbooks.htm

21   AVERT (2003) *Gay and Lesbian Information: homophobia and prejudice and attitudes to lesbians and gays.* AVERT. www.avert.org/hsexu3.htm

22   Department of Health (2001) *The Children Act 1989: guidance and regulations. Residential care. Vol. 4.* HMSO, London.

23   Social Exclusion Unit (2003) *A Better Education for Children in Care.* HMSO, London.

24   Hobcraft J (1998) *Intergenerational and Life Course Transmission of Social Exclusion: influences of childhood poverty, family disruption and involvement with the police.* Case paper 15. London School of Economics, London.

25   Biehal N, Clayden J, Stein M *et al.* (1992) *Prepared for Living? A survey of young people leaving the care of local authorities.* National Children's Bureau, London.

26   Biehal N, Clayden J, Stein M *et al.* (1995) *Moving On.* National Children's Bureau, London.

27   Department of Health (2000) *Children looked after at 31 March 1999 by placement and age.* DoH, London. www.doh.gov.uk/public/cla/tab_i.pdf

28   MacLeod M (1999) The abuse of children in institutional settings: children's perspectives. In: Stanley N, Manthorpe J and Penhale J (eds) *Institutional Abuse Perspectives Across the Life Course*, pp. 44–9. Routledge, London.

29   Blatt E (1992) Factors associated with child abuse and neglect in residential care settings. *Children and Youth Service Review.* **14**: 493–517.

30   Rosenthal J, Motz J, Edmonson D *et al.* (1991) A descriptive study of abuse and neglect in out-of-home placement. *Child Abuse and Neglect: the International Journal.* **15**: 249–60.

31   Sinclair I and Gibbs I (1998) *Children's Homes: a study in diversity.* Wiley, Chichester.

32   Waterhouse R (2000) *Lost in Care: report of the tribunal of inquiry into the abuse of children in care in the former county council areas of Gwynedd and Clwyd since 1974.* HMSO, London.

33 Quality Protects (1998) *Transforming Children's Services*. HMSO, London.
34 The Children's Society, NCH, NSPCC, Barnardo's and ECPAT UK (2002) *More Than One Chance*.
35 http://news.bbc.co.uk/1/hi/uk/1462628.stm
36 Barnardo's (1998) *Whose Daughter Next? Children Abused Through Prostitution*. Barnardo's, Ilford.
37 Department of Health (2002) *Safeguarding Children Involved in Prostitution: supplementary guidance to working together to safeguard children*. HMSO, London.
38 Department of Health and Association of Chief Police Officers (2002) *Children Missing From Care and From Home: a guide to good practice*. HMSO, London.
39 Department of Health (1999) *Working Together to Safeguard Children*. HMSO, London.

Resources

Ethnic groups

*   Blake S and Katrak Z (2002) *Faith, Values and SRE*. National Children's Bureau, London. www.ncb.org.uk/resources Book exploring faith and values and how they influence SRE.

*   Teenage Pregnancy Unit (2001) *Guidance for Developing Contraception and Sexual Health Advice Services to Reach Black and Minority Ethnic (BME) Young People*. HMSO, London. www.teenagepregnancyunit.gov.uk

*   Thompson R (ed) (1993) *Religion, Ethnicity and Sex Education: exploring the issues*. Sex Education Forum, National Children's Bureau, London. www.ncb.org.uk/resources

*   Teenage Pregnancy Unit (2002) *Diverse Communities: identity and teenage pregnancy*. HMSO, London. www.info.doh.gov.uk A project commissioned by the Teenage Pregnancy Unit to gather views via consultation with a variety of groups and individuals to develop a practical resource for making teenage pregnancy work more relevant and accessible to diverse communities.

Young men

*   Blake S and Laxton J (1998) *Strides*. Family Planning Association. A practical guide to sex and relationships education with young men.
    Available from the Family Planning Association (fpa) direct: PO Box 1078, East Oxford DO, Oxford OX4 6JS. Tel: 01865 719418. www.fpa.org.uk

*   www.youngfathers.org.uk
    Young Fathers Inc. offers services to young fathers in Croydon and Lewisham. These include advice sessions, an expectant fathers' course and a course for

young fathers with children of two and under. It provides recorded information on parental responsibility and the Child Support Agency (CSA) on 020 8760 5747, and offers help with sorting out disputes between young fathers and the mothers of their children. Leaflets and booklets containing information and advice for young fathers are also available. Tel: 020 8694 0812.

- Sex Education Forum (1997) *Supporting the Needs of Boys and Young Men in Sex and Relationships Education.* Factsheet 11. National Children's Bureau, London. www.ncb.org.uk/resources

Young people with disabilities

- *Cathy Has Thrush*
  Period Problems: what you can do
  Pictorial books for people with learning difficulties on women's health, promoting informed choices.
  Available from Women's Health, The Elfrida Society. Tel: 020 7251 6333. www.elfrida.com/publ.html

- McCarthy M and Thompson D (1992) *Sex and the 3 Rs: rights, responsibilities and risks. A sex education package for working with people with learning difficulties.* Pavilion Publishing, Brighton.

- *The Lyric*
  A video exploring issues around physical disability.
  Available from www.spod-uk.org/resources/video.html

- Scott L (1999) *Talking Together About Growing Up.* Pavilion Publishing, Brighton. Book providing support on subjects such as the life cycle, body parts, keeping safe, feelings, growing up and looking ahead for parents and carers of children with learning disabilities.

- *Kylie's Private World*
  A video for females with learning disabilities in support of general sex education, with strong emphasis on consent and how to say 'no'. First periods and sanitary protection and the use of condoms for safer sex are also explained.
  Available from www.lifesupportproductions.co.uk

- *Jason's Private World*
  A video for males with learning disabilities in support of general sex education, with strong emphasis on consent and how to both say 'no' and understand when someone else says 'no'. Also emphasised is the use of condoms for safe sex.
  Available from www.lifesupportproductions.co.uk

- *You, Your Body and Sex*
  An animated sex education video for people with learning disabilities. In trigger format for group discussion, it comes with an extensive information pack and viewing notes for carers.
  Available from www.lifesupportproductions.co.uk

Lesbian, gay, bisexual and transgender young people

- *Young Gay Men Talking*
  A leaflet featuring accounts from young gay men, including their coming to terms with their sexuality, coming out and their experiences of talking about their feelings with friends and parents, as well as their expectations, concerns and the realities of relationships with other gay men.
  Downloadable from www.avert.org/ypbooks.htm

- Forrest S, Biddle G and Clift S (2003) *Talking About Homosexuality in the Secondary School*. www.avert.org/ypbooks.htm Homosexuality is a subject that should be more widely discussed in schools. This book is a practical resource which should enable any school to make progress in this difficult area. It provides background information about homosexuality, the steps schools need to take before discussing the issues and strategies for talking about homosexuality with governors, parents, staff and students.

Looked-after children

- Mackie S and Patel-Kanwal H (2003) *Sex and Relationships Education for Young People in Care: let's make it happen.* Family Planning Association and National Children's Bureau, London.
  A training manual that enables trainers working in a range of settings to provide courses on sex, relationships, pregnancy and parenthood for professionals working with children and young people in care.
  Available from the fpa direct: PO Box 1078, East Oxford DO, Oxford OX4 6JS. Tel: 01865 719418. www.fpa.org.uk

- Social Exclusion Unit (2003) *A Better Education for Children in Care*. HMSO, London. www.socialexclusionunit.gov.uk

- Sex Education Forum (1998) *Talking About Sex and Relationships with Children and Young People in Public Care*. Forum Factsheet 17. National Children's Bureau, London. www.ncb.org.uk/resources

Children involved in prostitution

- Department of Health (2000) *Safeguarding Children Involved in Prostitution: supplementary guidance to working together to safeguard children. Quality protects.* HMSO, London. www.doh.gov.uk/scg/qualitycp.htm

CHAPTER 9

Setting up a young person's clinic

The vision for setting up a young person's clinic usually arises from a growing awareness of a gap in services. City and Hackney Young People's Services (*see* Chapter 7 for a summary of CHYPS work) have recently set up a sexual health clinic for young people in partnership with the local hospital sexual health department. It was through setting up this clinic that the idea for this book arose. The team working on the clinic had to do much research, planning and policy writing: the book brings this information together as a reference for other organisations in a similar position. This chapter provides a comprehensive check-list of the processes required to set up a clinic.

First, it is wise to consider whether it is best to set up a specific service for young people or to increase the youth friendliness of existing services. This can be decided by consulting with clients and staff and assessing what is practicable with the space, time and staff available. Similar processes will be required for both: mapping existing services, staff training, policy writing (the main ones being confidentiality and child protection), drawing up an operational policy and referral pathways, and considering how suitable the service and environment are for young people.

A survey of 'looked-after children', conducted by the Teenage Pregnancy Unit, elicited the following general recommendations concerning services provided for young people (*see* Box 9.1).[1] It is helpful to use this as a guide when considering the shape of a new project.

For those wishing to improve an existing general service for young people, McPherson *et al.* have produced an excellent book entitled *Healthcare of Young People: promotion in primary care.*[2] It provides useful information to help the primary healthcare team meet young people's needs. The top ten tips for 'getting it right for teenagers' are paraphrased as follows:

1   Organise a whole-team meeting to look at ways to improve the teen-friendliness of the service. Have you provided youth-friendly posters and leaflets, a confidentiality policy and a child protection policy?
2   Identify the characteristics of the 10–18 year-olds attending the service, e.g. gender, age; with this information services can be tailored to their needs.
3   Train appropriate staff members in contraception. This includes non-medical or nursing staff who may need training in interacting with young people. Ensure that your service has clear information stating that contraception is available to young people, including emergency contraception.

Box 9.1   Best practice guidance[1]

Any services provided for young people should:

- be accessible for individuals and small (mixed and single-sex) groups
- involve young people in providing advice and support
- ensure honesty
- ensure confidentiality
- be in relaxed environments where young people feel at ease and are with others in similar situations
- be fun, creative and easy to use
- be flexible – operating after school, in the evenings, at weekends or via drop-ins so that they can be accessed when young people feel they need support
- present information in accessible, interesting and humorous ways
- provide advice about available options, how to access services, what to expect and additional sources of support
- include general information and advice from specialists
- include transport, if necessary
- include child care for young parents.

---

4   Inform young people exactly what the service provides. Develop a service information booklet for them.
5   Focus on confidentiality. Ensure that there is publicity emphasising the fact that the service is confidential for under-16s. Look at staff members' knowledge of confidentiality issues; is any training required?
6   Advertise services that are available for young people outside your service.
7   Consider organising a separate young person's clinic; would this be beneficial and practicable?
8   Consider involving parents. During teen years parents are still the main providers of health information for young people. Could you support them in this by providing information, sessions and resources?
9   Offer advice and support for teens who do get pregnant.
10 Ensure that young men are considered in all aspects.

The young person's clinic

When setting up a specific young person's clinic, the first step is to identify the needs of the community and map out existing services. Investigate other interested parties as there might be a possibility of partnership working. The 'one-stop shop' concept (one clinic that provides several services such as sexual health, contraception, counselling, and alcohol and drug counselling) is advocated in the Government's National Strategy for Sexual Health and HIV.[3] It is popular with young people as they can access information on a variety of issues at once; and, when seeking contraceptive and sexual health advice, it is not obvious that this is what they are doing. A study from the USA found that young people attending specialist youth clinics which provided medical, social and mental health services had a wider range of problems detected than those attending the usual primary healthcare facilities.[4]

If you do decide to work in partnership with another organisation, it is important to share a philosophy and clear working relations. It might be an idea to produce a handbook that outlines the service philosophy, people's contact details, and the terms and conditions of the project. This handbook would also contain the operational policy, general policies for practice, staff roles and responsibilities, and care and referral pathways.

Consulting young people

Article 12 of the United Nations Convention on the Rights of the Child,[5] ratified by the UK in 1991, established the right of young people to be consulted and listened to by public service providers. Before setting up a young person's service it is vital to consult with young people, as only then will services be tailored to their needs. Ideally, young people should be involved in all decision-making processes, including planning, organisation, staffing, funding, management, delivery, evaluation and dissemination. Once a service is set up there should be independent, accessible mechanisms for young people to register complaints, provide feedback and make suggestions about improving services.[6]

A range of qualitative and quantitative methods can be used to elicit young people's opinions: questionnaires, interviews, focus groups and stakeholder conferences. Box 9.2 contains an example of how drama was used in conjunction with peer interviewing to elicit and present young people's views on healthcare services.[7]

Participatory approaches to consultation are recommended as they empower participants to identify their own issues and priorities. The process of involvement

---

Box 9.2   'Follow the Fish': involving young people in primary care in Midlothian[7]

Aims
The aims of the project were to enable young people to contribute their views about health services, to encourage professionals and policy makers to listen to young people and to stimulate action to address the issues raised.

Design
Peer interviews were undertaken by a team of five young people to identify the experiences and views of young people about health services. Drama workshop sessions were conducted with young people; these encompassed initial issue-identifying activities and group discussion about their own experiences of, and views about, health services. They were followed by role play and improvisation to construct drama scenarios about the issues gathered from the interviews and discussions.

Twenty young people aged 12–16 years took part in the project. The project was conducted as a voluntary after-school activity for 12 weeks.

Results

A drama was constructed from the young people's research and performed by them to an invited audience of 30 health and education professionals. A post-performance question and answer session was then held with the audience to explore the issues raised.

Conclusions

Drama can offer a means to encourage participation, facilitate participants' self-expression and explore health/health service themes and issues. In conjunction with conventional techniques such as interviews and group discussions, a drama project can also be used to communicate the experiences, views and needs of the wider client group to service providers and planners. Such initiatives may generate outcomes to improve service users' experiences of health services.

Cast members made the following comments after the performance:

'The play gave us a good way to get our message across. Reports on a sheet of paper are easy to ignore, but with the drama we could act how we felt, how we get treated and how we want to be treated.'

'We think the play will get across to the authorities and hopefully some of them will talk to colleagues so that things are made better for young people.'

should be made enjoyable in order to create interest and engage young people. Good practice would include methods where young people can play an active role, such as peer interviewing and discussion workshops.[7]

Establishing a working party

Once it is decided who will be involved in the project, a working party should be established. This should be made up of a representative from each body involved and with young people represented. With several factions involved, the project may progress more slowly; however, workload is easier as it can be shared and different views on a project will make for a more rounded service.

In the working party, brainstorm your ideas for the project. What are its aims and objectives? Are they realistic? What will the project achieve and how? All involved should be clear on the project goals; once the service is up and running, outcomes can be measured against the objectives. Having clear objectives makes evaluation easier and bids for funding and extra staff etc. will be more forthcoming with tangible results.

In your working party note down all the resources you will need. Consider financial, material and human resources. Who will you need, what will be their roles, who do you have available and for how long? What material resources do you need? A venue, equipment, monies, literature?

Box 9.3   Bodyzone in Oxfordshire[9]

In Oxfordshire, Bodyzone clinics have been set up in 16 secondary schools, providing a comprehensive health information, advice and support service for young people. They are staffed by a school health nurse, family planning nurse and youth worker, with back-up from a local GP.

A community-based Bodyzone service is also being developed to provide the service out of school hours and during holidays in order to include young people not attending school. This is a joint initiative between the Teenage Pregnancy Partnership Board, Sure Start, school health nursing teams and the youth service.[9]

Where will the clinic be located?

The clinic should be located in a place that is accessible and appealing to young people (*see* Box 9.3). While hospitals and surgeries may have the facilities required, their clinical nature is not always appealing to young people. This was illustrated by a study that showed that when clients aged under 25 years who attended a London Brook service were referred to GUM clinics, only 17% attended. Attendance was much higher at a young person's clinic.[8] Consider less orthodox settings where young people can be found, such as schools, shopping centres, sports complexes, etc. For example, a mobile contraceptive and sexual health clinic in North Staffordshire enables young people to access services in non-traditional settings such as youth clubs and sports facilities.[9]

Once you have several options for the clinic location, consider the space available. Is there appropriate space for filing cabinets, sufficient reception space, seating, and enough clinical rooms with the appropriate furniture and equipment? Is security required? A full risk assessment will highlight any areas for change or improvement or indicate that it is not a suitable venue.

Risk assessment consists of five steps:

1 look for hazards
2 decide who might be harmed and how
3 evaluate the risks and decide whether the existing precautions are adequate or whether more should be done
4 record your findings
5 review your assessment and revise if necessary.

For a more detailed description of risk assessment, the following website from NHS Plus is useful: www.nhsplus.nhs.uk/Law&you/employers_riskassessment.asp

The environment

The service atmosphere should be welcoming to young people. As young people's services are often on a drop-in basis, they can spend a good deal of time waiting to be seen. Often young people find services cold, clinical and unfriendly. How can the environment be made more welcoming to young people? Is the service easily accessible and clearly signposted? Who are they likely to come into contact with when accessing the clinic? Are these people welcoming to young people? Once at the clinic, is the waiting room comfortable? What are the chairs like? Is it possible to provide refreshments? Are there children's toys? Could there be music or TV provided? As well as silence in the waiting room being uncomfortable, it also has implications for confidentiality when all waiting can hear the conversations between receptionist and client (*see* Chapter 2 for discussion on young people and the clinic environment).

What is the best time for the clinic?

The consultation with young people will indicate what is the preferred time for the clinic. However, a preferred time may not be a practical time, hence a survey of other successful clinics and times will aid decision making. Popular times are after-school clinics where young people can attend before they are expected home or Saturdays (usually in the afternoon). If the clinic is in a non-traditional setting such as a college or school, a time during the day may be suitable.

Staffing

What staff will you need to cover all aspects of the clinic: medical, nursing, counsellors, health advisers, personal advisers, administrative, reception? The responsibilities of each staff member should be clear, as well as the boundaries to their roles.

For a smooth referral system, relations should be set up with relevant agencies and communication pathways put in place. It should be clear who will be responsible for any follow-up. Often staff for individual clinics are drawn from other services and follow-up can get forgotten or it is assumed that others are pursuing it.

Are there any training issues? Are all staff aware of young people's issues? Are they young people-friendly? Will they be non-judgemental and listen to clients? Staff, including any volunteers or trainees, may require training about young people's needs and appropriate strategies for working with them. Do they need training that gives them the opportunity to explore their attitudes to young people and sexuality?

Are all staff aware of relevant policies such as record keeping, confidentiality, data protection and child protection? Are they aware of legislation, guidance and research findings concerning their area of work, and available local/regional/national services or sources of information such as:

- The Children Act 1989[10]
- Teenage Pregnancy Strategy[11]
- National Strategy for Sexual Health and HIV[3]
- Sexual Offences Act (2003)[12]
- Working Together to Safeguard Children.[13]

If working in partnership with other organisations, which policies and procedures will you adopt and who will be responsible for ensuring they are kept up to date?

Are there clear clinical supervision (*see* Appendix 7 for the background and definition of clinical supervision) and staff support mechanisms? Is there opportunity for staff to voice concerns and worries? For a comprehensive guide to clinical supervision, the following website is useful: www.clinical-supervision.com

How will the clinic be run?

It is useful to have an overall operational policy that sets out staff responsibilities and includes all relevant policies. More specialised services may need to consider developing additional policies specific to the clinic, such as pregnancy testing and condom provision.

Child protection and confidentiality will be key issues for any young person's clinic. The tool-kit on confidentiality and young people developed by the Royal College of General Practitioners and Brook is an excellent resource and provides sample confidentiality policy agreements that can be adapted for individual clinics.[14]

The confidentiality policy should clearly set out:

- the importance of confidentiality
- that clients are entitled to a confidential service, including those aged under 16
- that professional codes of conduct and employment contracts require confidentiality to be maintained by all those working in the clinic.

People who are not employed directly by the practice but who are working in the surgery (including students, volunteers or anyone observing practice) should also be given a copy.

A sample confidentiality policy has been adapted from the RCGP/Brook confidentiality tool-kit[14] and included as Appendix 8. A sample child protection policy is included as Appendix 9 and can be built upon and customised to the service provided.

Referral pathways

Young people may need referring on to other agencies for support in areas not provided by the clinic. It is important to have clear referral pathways to ensure rapid follow-up. The operational policy should include referral criteria and contacts for: child protection, drug and alcohol support services, social services, young families support service, midwifery, a paediatrician, police, a looked-after children nurse specialist, and any other relevant professionals.

Care pathways

The operational policy can include care pathways and assessment pro formas for common scenarios encountered within the clinic. This ensures a service standard within the team and documentation that can be audited in the evaluation process. A definition of an integrated care pathway is found in Appendix 10. Further information regarding integrated care pathways can be found on the National electronic Library for Health website at the following address: www.nelh.uk/ carepathways/

Advertising the service

Naming the service

It must be remembered that the name of a service suggests the nature of its clients. One study found the term 'family planning' off-putting for young people (family planning implying that the service is aimed at older couples who are planning a family):

> You don't think people your age would go to the family planning clinic? Not yet, not until we started family planning ... settling down – that's when you're planning.

In the same study, young people associated GUM services with dentistry![15]

Publicity methods

Be creative – as well as leaflets and posters, consider other publicity methods. For example, wallet-sized cards with information about services are popular. They are easy for young people to take away, particularly if placed in discreet areas such as public toilets. Consider adverts on local radio stations and at clubs.

Designing the style and content of promotional material

Promotional material should match the standards of style-conscious consumer advertising and be both fashionable and eye-catching. Health promotion material should steer clear of messages that are too negative yet highlight sexual health risks. Use of humour is appealing to young people, as are contemporary images. Care is needed when using images of young people as it may convey particular messages. For example, a single male may suggest the service is for homosexuals; too 'couply' and it might suggest it is for established couples only. Publicity will be more effective if young people are involved in its creation and design.

Locating the material

There are two types of location where services can be advertised: places where a young person will actively seek information on a service, e.g. GP surgeries, health centres; and passive locations where a young person is inadvertently exposed to promotional material, e.g. shopping centres, college, hoardings, etc. In both scenarios the young person needs to be able to view the material discreetly and confidentially.

Representation at a strategic level

It is important that the service is represented at a strategic level. Ensure that it is being promoted at board level; this will disseminate information about your service and secure support and funding.

Evaluation/review

Evaluation measures need to be in place from the start to assess the work's impact and to inform service development. Evaluation is essential to good project management. It answers questions such as:

- Did the project achieve its goals?
- Was the project successful?
- What worked and why?
- What didn't work and why?
- How can the project be improved?
- What has been learned that can inform others?

There are three possible goals to evaluation:

1 to judge the project's success
2 to provide feedback to inform the ongoing direction of a project
3 to generate or enhance knowledge of a particular subject area. This type of evaluation is not expected to directly influence the assessment or direction of a project but to influence thinking in general (usually conducted in universities by academics).

Evaluation can take place at the beginning of a project and is part of the needs assessment, risk assessment and general consultative process; there can also be evaluation during the project, which asks questions such as:

- Is the project progressing according to plan?
- Are key stakeholders engaged?
- Are the anticipated benefits being realised?
- Are any new benefits emerging?
- What are the key barriers faced and how can they be overcome?

Finally, evaluation at the end of a project asks:

- Did the project achieve its goals?
- Are the stakeholders satisfied with the outcome?
- What were the main achievements?
- What are the key lessons learned and recommendations for further work?

Both staff and clients should be asked to evaluate the service. In order to ensure that problems are solved and staff have the opportunity to voice any concerns, there should be regular staff feedback reviews.

Young people's opinions of the service should also be sought. A range of evaluation tools can be used, including focus group discussion, questionnaires and surveys.

Summary

Use the following as a check-list when improving or setting up a specific service for young people. If making an existing service more youth-friendly, consider the following:

☐ Hold a team meeting.
☐ Brainstorm possible improvements to the service.
☐ Posters/leaflets.
☐ Confidentiality policy; publicise confidentiality.
☐ Child protection policy.
☐ Carry out a profile for young people in your service.
☐ Staff training.
☐ Have clear specific information for young people.
☐ Advertise other young people's services in the area.
☐ Support parents in communicating health messages to their children.
☐ Consider young men in all aspects.

For a specific service consider the following:

☐ Identify community needs; map out existing services.
☐ Network with other like-minded groups and individuals.
☐ Consider working in partnership.
☐ Consult with young people.
☐ Establish a working party. Set out aims and objectives and how to achieve these. List resources required; consider financial, material and human resources.
☐ Organise any training required.
☐ Where will the service be located? It needs to be accessible and welcoming to young people and appropriate for the service provided.
☐ Carry out a risk assessment for the proposed location.
☐ Consider the clinic environment; is it young people-friendly?
☐ What time will the clinic be held?
☐ Write an operational policy and include the following:

- if working in partnership, write a shared philosophy and terms and conditions
- draw up staff roles and responsibilities
- draw up referral pathways
- write policies
- write care pathways.

☐ Advertise the service:

- choose an appealing name
- be creative when promoting the service
- involve young people in the design and style of publicity material
- use humour and images
- consider effective locations for publicity materials
- advertise your service at a strategic level.

☐ Evaluate the project.
☐ Involve both staff and clients in evaluation.

References

1 Teenage Pregnancy Unit (2000) *Best Practice Guidance on the Provision of Effective Contraception and Advice Service for Young People.* HMSO, London.
2 McPherson A, Donovan C and Macfarlane A (2002) *Healthcare of Young People: promotion in primary care.* Radcliffe Medical Press, Oxford.
3 Department of Health (2000) *National Strategy for Sexual Health and HIV.* HMSO, London.
4 Earls F, Robins LEN, Stiffman AR *et al.* (1989) Comprehensive health care for high-risk adolescents: an evaluation study. *American Journal of Public Health.* **79**: 999–1005.
5 www.unicef.org.uk/education/whatisCRC.htm
6 Teenage Pregnancy Unit (2001) *A Guide to Involving Young People in Teenage Pregnancy Work.* HMSO, London.
7 Jackson AM (2003) 'Follow the Fish': involving young people in primary care in Midlothian. *Health Expectations.* **6**: 342–51.
8 Vanhegan G and Wedgewood A (1999) A young people's understanding of safer sex and their attitude to referral for STI screening: two audits from London Brook Advisory Centres. *British Journal of Family Planning.* **25**: 22–4.
9 www.doh.gov.uk/cmo/progress/inequalities/teenage.htm
10 Department for Education and Skills (1989) *The Children Act 1989.* HMSO, London.
11 Social Exclusion Unit (1999) *Teenage Pregnancy Strategy.* HMSO, London.
12 Home Office (2003) *Sexual Offences Act 2003.* HMSO, London.
13 Department of Health (1999) *Working Together to Safeguard Children.* HMSO, London.
14 Royal College of General Practitioners and Brook (2000) *Confidentiality and Young People: improving teenagers' uptake of sexual and other health advice. A toolkit for general practice, primary care groups and trusts.* RCGP and Brook, London.
15 Pearson S (2003) Promoting sexual health services to young men: findings from focus group discussions. *Journal of Family Planning and Reproductive Health Care.* **29** (4): 194–8.

Resources
Service provision

• Teenage Pregnancy Unit (2000) *Best Practice Guidance on the Provision of Effective Contraception and Advice Service for Young People.* HMSO, London. www.teenagepregnancyunit.gov.uk

• McPherson A, Donovan C and Macfarlane A (2002) *Healthcare of Young People: promotion in primary care.* Radcliffe Medical Press, Oxford.

- Sex Education Forum (2001) *Working with Young People in Sexual Health Settings: a provider's guide.* Factsheet 25. National Children's Bureau, London. www.ncb. org.uk/sexed.htm

Confidentiality

See Chapter 3 for further resources on confidentiality.

Consultation

- Cohen J and Emanuel J (1998) *Positive Participation: consulting and involving young people in health-related work. A planning and training resource.* Health Education Authority, London.

- Save the Children (2001) *Re-action Consultation Tool-kit.* Save the Children, Scotland.

- Teenage Pregnancy Unit (2001) *A Guide to Involving Young People in Teenage Pregnancy Work.* HMSO, London. www.teenagepregnancyunit.gov.uk

CHAPTER 10

Sexual health outreach in youth settings

What is outreach?

Outreach work involves accessing young people and providing them with information to make informed decisions about their sexual health. Sex and relationships education (SRE) delivered throughout a young person's life through school, that provides clear and unambiguous information, is effective in changing knowledge and attitudes.[1] Evidence has shown that programmes in schools designed to increase young people's knowledge about sexual health, self-esteem and decision-making skills lead to delayed sexual intercourse; if intercourse does occur, the couple are more likely to use a condom.[2] It is reasonable to suppose that programmes in community settings would have a similar outcome.

SRE outreach by community professionals

Workshops by community professionals in schools and youth settings can introduce several professional adults who can fulfil a supportive role for young people. It is valuable to have a range of professionals involved in delivering SRE so that students are offered a wide choice of people with whom they can discuss different issues of concern. In addition, outreach work by community professionals links young people into community services.

This chapter deals with outreach in all youth settings; however, much can be learned from the work that has been done around SRE in schools. In the light of recent teenage pregnancy and sexual health figures there has been much attention to the content of SRE in schools: when to start teaching sex education, what should be taught, how and by whom. The National Curriculum gives guidance on recommended teaching at each age and is a useful and legal framework around which other professionals can base their SRE teaching.

Outreach in schools

Often community groups are invited into schools to provide sessions on an aspect of sexual health. This has many benefits: it provides young people with sexual health information and negotiation skills, links young people into community services, introduces professionals who work in the community, and provides support for teaching staff.

When working in schools, community professionals may find that the school is part of a scheme called the National Healthy School Standard (*see* Appendix 11 for details). This provides a framework for a whole-school approach to health and includes standards that relate to the delivery of effective SRE. Whether part of the Healthy School Standard or not, a school should have an SRE policy and programme that visiting professionals should be shown to inform their work.

Content of SRE curriculum

The SRE curriculum for key stages 3 and 4 (secondary school level) is a useful guide for pitching outreach work in schools. To view the full National Curriculum, visit www.nc.uk.net.

The personal, social and health education (PSHE) and citizenship framework provides a planning tool for holistic provision of SRE. The biological content of sex education is laid out in the National Science Curriculum and is supplemented with the social, moral and emotional aspects of sex education in *Curriculum Guidance 5: health education*.[3] The Education Act 1996[4] requires all maintained secondary schools to provide a sex education curriculum that includes teaching about HIV/AIDS and STIs. (At primary level the governing body decides whether to provide additional sex education beyond that provided by the National Curriculum.) An extract from the National Curriculum that sets out the curriculum content pertaining to SRE for secondary schools is included in Appendix 12.

A summary follows:

- Both boys and girls should be prepared for puberty.
- Young people need access to, and precise information about, confidential contraceptive information, advice and services.
- Young people need to be aware of the moral and personal dilemmas involved in abortion and know how to access a relevant agency if necessary.
- Young people need to be aware of the risks of STIs, including HIV, and know about prevention, diagnosis and treatment.
- Young people need to know not just what safer sex is and why it is important, but also how to negotiate it with a partner.

SRE is lifelong learning about sex, sexuality, emotions, relationships and sexual health. It involves acquiring accurate information, developing skills, positive values and a moral framework that will guide decision making, judgements and behaviour.[5] The Sex Education Forum (National Children's Bureau) describes sex education as having three elements: the acquisition of information; the development of social skills; and the development of moral responsibility and values.[6] This is a good framework to bear in mind when doing outreach work in schools or youth organisations.

Planning your outreach

Groundwork

Once a session is proposed and accepted within a community organisation, it is helpful to have a clear process to work through to ensure that the host organisation and provider have a clear understanding of what is being provided. The host organisation needs to know who is visiting their organisation, their philosophy, what the sessions will cover and any appropriate feedback. The outreach team need to know what is required of them, who they will be working with, host organisation policies and their evaluation after the workshop. This will involve meeting with the host organisation (perhaps more than once, depending on the complexity of the outreach work proposed), planning, delivering and evaluating the session.

Meet with the host organisation

It is important to meet with the host organisation before the session. There should be a named contact with whom you decide what work will be carried out and its aims, and who needs to be involved, consulted and informed. This contact person can provide the visitor with copies of relevant organisation policies. It is useful for both parties to have a contract where roles, responsibilities and boundaries are clearly outlined.

This contract should include:

- who is going to be carrying out the sessions
- what is going to be covered in the sessions
- the named contact in the school
- the role of teaching and support staff
- statements regarding child protection and confidentiality
- statements regarding bullying
- the procedure if a young person leaves the session
- a commitment to evaluation and feedback.

Confidentiality

It is generally agreed that a visitor to a classroom should work within the school confidentiality policy in classroom sessions, but can work within their professional guidelines when working individually with pupils. If working in a youth organisation, check their confidentiality policy for any variations to this approach.

Child protection policy/procedures

Every institution should have a policy for dealing with disclosure of sexual abuse, together with referral procedures. Many professionals feel unskilled in dealing with a personal disclosure of a sensitive nature. It is helpful to be prepared and anticipate what to do and say in such a situation. On-the-spot strategies for dealing with disclosure or an explicit question that raises concerns about sexual abuse include:

- React calmly and acknowledge that you have heard what the young person has said and that you think it is important.
- Tell them it sounds like something you should talk about after the session and in a private place.

- Make sure you do talk to them afterwards, accept what they tell you and tell them what the procedure is, e.g. it could be that a social worker needs to be involved.

Involving parents

Before launching into a programme for young people it is worth considering how to involve parents. Young people cite parents as their preferred source of sex and relationships information; however, parents often feel ill-equipped to provide this information. A survey of parents by the Sex Education Forum showed:[7]

- there is a general lack of guidance for parents on how best to approach sex education at home
- they would like suggestions of appropriate books/booklets to use with their children
- they would like assistance with age appropriateness of topics and guidance on the depth of information to provide
- they value material to support sex education
- they would like support with particular topics, including contraception, homosexuality, abortion, HIV/AIDS and supporting young people to delay sex
- they would like to be consulted over the subjects to be covered in school, the ages at which these subjects are taught and the style of delivery.

If it is a school programme, parents should always be informed that visitors are attending the school to participate in the SRE curriculum and of the programme content. Parents have the right to withdraw their children from SRE classes but not from those that cover the curriculum content: namely STIs and contraception. Check how the school is informing parents of your involvement in the curriculum. Perhaps they could include your organisation's leaflet and contact details in case parents have any questions. Informative leaflets on the subjects you will be covering in the session(s) could also be sent out.

For parents who want to become more actively involved in their child's SRE, resources and books could be made available and appropriate materials suggested. There could be a series of workshops with parents, covering areas where they would like more information. There may also be the possibility of creative programmes such as parents being trained as peer educators and providing SRE guidance for other parents. Box 10.1 contains an example of a parent peer education programme in Sheffield. It has been summarised from a full description on the Sheffield Centre for HIV and Sexual Health website.[8]

Box 10.1 Sheffield Centre for HIV and Sexual Health: Parent-to-Parent Project[8]

Summary
The Parent-to-Parent Project is a parent peer education group. Parents are trained to run sex education sessions for other parents in community settings in Sheffield. The aim is to build parents' confidence to have honest and open discussions with their children and thereby increase their children's

knowledge of sexual and reproductive health. Studies reveal that although parents want sex education to be provided in schools, they feel they have a major role to play in the sex and sexual health education of their children.

Project description
- The project aims to increase children's and young people's sexual health awareness by increasing parents' confidence and skills on how to talk about sex through recruiting and training a group of 14 peer educators. The project is coordinated on a voluntary basis by three parents from the original project, and overseen by the Sheffield Centre for HIV and Sexual Health. The training of new groups of peer educators is undertaken by the Project Coordinator and Project Leader from the first phase. A recruitment flyer, mailing, press release and word of mouth are all used to reach potential trainees.
- The volunteer training course consists of experiential and participative sessions. The modules of the course cover team building, values review, language, communicating, group work skills, presentation and facilitation skills, organising a session and evaluation.
- Since completing the training, the peer educators have run one-off sex education sessions with other parents in primary and secondary schools, GP surgeries, voluntary organisations and family centres. These are friendly and informal sessions of about two hours, during which the peer educators use a range of participative exercises to encourage parents to share experiences and learn from each other about how to communicate with their children.

Achievements
There is evidence that the training can be a transformational and empowering process for the peer educators and parents attending sessions. It builds the confidence of attendees, increases their sexual health knowledge and ability to communicate openly about sex with their children.

Assessing your group

It is vital to gather as much information as possible about the group prior to planning and delivering a session. What is the group size? Are there any special needs or circumstances? How many facilitators are required? Do you require male and female facilitators? When asked, young people said the gender of the sex educator was not an issue, although boys do express a wish for a male facilitator at least some of the time – someone who can empathise with their feelings and worries.[9]

If possible, meet with the young people before the work is carried out. Ask them what they want from the sessions. This will give you an idea of group dynamics and the opportunity to tailor the session to their needs.

Consult with young people, parents and teachers to ensure that sessions are inclusive of different faiths and cultures. Outreach will need to be flexible, e.g. sometimes providing single-gender lessons where appropriate to ensure that young people's faiths are respected. Consultation with parents and young people will ensure that practice is not based on stereotypes and false assumptions.

Visit the venue prior to taking the session. It is important that the venue for the workshop is carefully chosen to promote a positive atmosphere. Is there enough space? Does the space enable free and safe movement? Does it allow for confidentiality? Will you be able to use any audiovisual equipment? Is it comfortable, warm and light?

Suggested activities

Once you know your group, location, time frame and desired content, the session itself can be planned. Young people learn in different ways and they will benefit most from outreach that uses a variety of teaching methods. Active learning is better received than didactic teaching as it uses creative processes to develop skills. Active participation in their own learning by young people increases the likelihood of the experience being meaningful, relevant and effective. They will benefit from hearing and exploring the diverse beliefs, values, opinions and feelings of others. Activities should provide them with the opportunity to explore issues and the space to look at their own values. In addition, a variety of learning experiences increases energy levels and interest, and communication skills, collaborative work and ideas are articulated and practised.

When planning an activity the following general questions will guide the choice of activities:[6]

- What are you trying to achieve?
- What activity will best achieve the outcome?
- What is the size of the group?
- How well do the young people in the group know each other?
- How well do you know the group?
- How familiar are the young people with informal learning methods?
- What are the different levels of ability of the group?
- What does the group already know?

The following are activity suggestions that can be worked into a session. All suggestions actively involve the young people, give the choice of working in a large group, small group or individually, and help them explore issues.

Brainstorming
Brainstorming allows the group to write down all thoughts without any censoring. It introduces the idea that there are no right nor wrong answers. Brainstorming provides a good starting point for discussing issues and ideas.

Pairs and small-group work
Working in pairs on a task or quiz is useful for working on sensitive or more personal issues. Similarly, small groups are safer than large groups, especially if sharing attitudes and values.

Scenarios
Work and discussion around a scenario can lead to exploration of attitudes, values and feelings. Using a situation that is similar to young people's experience without it being their own provides the opportunity to discuss personal issues.

Quizzes and questionnaires
Quizzes and questionnaires can trigger discussion, clarify information and allow facilitators to assess the group's knowledge.

Continuum
Continuums can be used to explore attitudes and values. Two opposing statements are put at different ends of the room and the young people are asked to stand between them depending on their opinion. Once in place the young people's beliefs and opinions can be explored.

Drama
Using drama is a good distancing technique. This can be in many forms, e.g. reading from diaries, letters, journals. These can be written as a means of reflecting on a character's experience or introduced by the facilitator as a piece of evidence or insight into a character's thoughts and feelings about a dilemma or experience.

Developing a character from a picture
A character (cartoon, well-known soap character, etc.) is presented in picture form. Information is then read or requested regarding a situation or dilemma for the young people to discuss.

Role play
An individual or group takes on a character role and responds to a situation. This technique allows young people to explore situations from a different perspective, to get feedback on how their message has been received and to practise skills, e.g. negotiating and communicating.

One variation on role play would be 'hot seating' a character. A group working as themselves have the opportunity to question or interview a person/people who are in character. This can highlight characters' experiences, feelings and motivations, and encourage insights into the relationship between attitudes and events, as well as an awareness of human behaviour.

Check-list for facilitators

Once you have devised a workshop, look at the structure, content and running time. Ask the following questions:

- Does the session relate to the individual's/group's experience?
- Have you allowed for different abilities in the group?
- Are you using simple yet creative activities?
- Are you clear why you are using these activities and how they fit in with your aims and objectives?
- Are they achievable in the time?
- Does the session relate to past and future work?
- Is it inclusive (for girls, boys, diverse ability, disability, sexual orientation, ethnic groups and belief systems)?
- Are you allowing the young people to reflect on their learning?
- Are you summarising at regular intervals? Do you use repetition and reinforcement of ideas/skills?
- Are you using props to illustrate concepts and ideas?

It is useful to set out the workshop in table format, including running times. This provides a template for planning future sessions and can be given as guidance to anybody assisting with the session. The following is an example of a contraception workshop devised for the City and Hackney SRE Team.[10]

SRE Workshop Plan

Title: Contraception

Venue:

Facilitators:

Date:

Aims: to raise awareness of the range of contraceptives available; to identify risk and difficult situations; to develop communication skills around contraception and asking for advice/support.

Learning outcomes: by the end of the session young people will be able to demonstrate an increased understanding of some of the methods and skills that can be used to avoid unwanted pregnancy and protect against STIs, and how to access support.

Time	Activity	Aim	Resources
5	**Introduction/welcome**		
5	**Icebreaker**: name game		
10	**Group agreement/** expectations of the session		Flip chart, paper, etc. or set expectations that group can agree with or add to.
5	1 **Setting the scene**: what is contraception? (a) what does word mean? 'contra' = 'against' and 'conception' = joining of egg and sperm, etc. (b) what do people do if they want to avoid having a baby? Verbal discussion with group.	To raise awareness of the range of contraceptives available. To identify myths. To develop communication about contraception.	

Time	Activity	Aim	Resources
10	2 Fact/fiction-type activity, e.g. what is or isn't a form of contraception in the box? Group takes turns to pick one out and say whether it is a form of contraception or not, and puts in two piles. Show range but not in-depth explanation at this stage. Write up the names of the types of contraception, and add others that young people know of. Discuss myths and misconceptions as they arise.		Box with hole in top for 'feel' activity, containing types of contraception and non-contraceptives, e.g. sponge, bubble bath, lemon, tampon, plastic bag, female condom, picture of person crossing their fingers, etc.
30	**Knowledge** (active learning): contraceptive methods activity. Keep to four commonly used contraceptives, e.g. pills, emergency contraception, condoms (male and female) 1 Stations are set up on different tables or areas, with an envelope and small box on each. 2 Small groups move round (5 mins on each) and look at the resources and write two questions they would like to know the answers to on the slips of paper. These are put in the box on the table. 3 Whole group back together. Facilitators take each box and ask young people to pull out a question, or facilitators do this. Ask group first if they know answers; facilitator clarifies and answers questions.	To allow young people to practise asking questions about things they want to know. To allow for opportunity for small-group discussion about contraception and to ask questions in written form they may feel shy/unable to ask verbally.	Envelopes containing a brief description and picture and/or sample of contraceptive method; four small boxes and blank slips of paper.

Time	Activity	Aim	Resources
20	Condom demonstration and practice: 1 condom demo by facilitators 2 practising in pairs on demonstrators	To practise how to put on and take off a condom.	Condoms (male and female); demonstrators.
	3 additional activity – rubbing oils into condoms after they are blown up to demonstrate how this perforates and weakens the condom.	To see how certain oils can weaken a condom.	Range of oils which should not be used with condoms, e.g. Vaseline, baby oil, cooking oil, massage oil.
10–15	**Skills and attitudes**: negotiation/communicating what you want activity. For example, saying 'no' in a round. (Facilitator in centre, throws ball to each group member in turn. They must then throw it back to the facilitator, saying 'no' with conviction!)	To identify difficult situations/different attitudes in negotiating condom use. To practise some of these skills in a safe way.	Ball.
	Drama – if time and level of confidence of facilitator permit. Role play/scenario negotiating condom use/ accessing condoms, etc.	To identify barriers to condom use/safer sex, internal and external factors (i.e. pressure, expectations, not wanting to be seen as easy, etc.).	
10	**Accessing services**: role play clinic visit/ pharmacy attendance to access emergency contraception.	To practise communication/ asking questions. To inform young people of procedures at clinics/what to expect.	

Time	Activity	Aim	Resources
10	Activity to check learning/ understanding/applying what they have learned in the session. Ideas: 1 use agony aunt type letters – someone reads out and group offers advice 2 a quiz 3 fact or fiction – individual sheets.	To check understanding/ learning and inform facilitators how session has gone.	Quiz sheets.
5	**Evaluation**: written forms/post-it notes, etc.		Post-it notes; flip-chart paper, pens.
5	Closing round. One thing they have got from session, etc. A calming activity before end.		

Delivery

To create a relaxed, safe environment it is helpful to create a group agreement at the beginning of the session. This allows group ownership of the session and forms the boundaries within which the group will be working. It is drawn up by the pupils with some guidance from the facilitators. It can include issues such as respect for others in the group, only one person to speak at a time, maintaining confidentiality, all mobile phones to be switched off, etc. In addition, it provides a useful tool to refer to if any of these issues arise during the session.

For young people to feel comfortable in a session they need to be reassured of confidentiality. Discuss this at the beginning of the session. Clarify that what is discussed in the session is confidential (this needs to be part of the group agreement) and explain your code of confidentiality: if approached on a one-to-one basis you can maintain confidentiality unless the young person or others are in danger (see Chapter 3 for further details); if in a group situation the teacher responsible for child protection will need to be informed. The activities in the session should use distancing techniques and realistic case studies rather than personal experience; this will help to protect confidentiality.

Throughout the session continually reflect on how well it is going and how the young people are responding to the activities. Be prepared to move on to another activity if the group is not responding or is flagging. Use open questioning, be clear about why you are using an activity, give clear instructions, be encouraging and be available to individuals within the group.

The challenge is not simply to impart knowledge, but also to manage the group. Continuously monitor the dynamics of the group and adapt the session as necessary. For example, if in small groups bring the group back together; consider an activity that requires the young people to work individually or a game to distract and rekindle enthusiasm, etc. Always allow for flexibility. Have more activities ready than you think you will need.

Facilitators are not expected to know everything, they are there to help and guide the young people. If a young person asks a question you do not know the answer to, be honest and ensure you find the answer for them or direct them to someone who will be able to provide the information.

A note on self-disclosure

Self-disclosure is never appropriate nor necessary. Although it may be tempting to illustrate the lesson with experiences from your own life, it is not good practice to share the details of your life and relationships. It might suggest that you expect the young people to do the same, which would be threatening and may lead to teasing and bullying. Role model how to discuss personal issues in an impersonal way, e.g. 'Sharon (in Eastenders) this week had to face the dilemma of ... how do you think she should resolve the situation?'

A note on bullying/homophobia

There is now clear recognition that emotional bullying, name calling and isolating individuals are as destructive to self-esteem as physical bullying. One particular form of bullying, homophobia, is common amongst young men. Young men can be particularly intolerant of different sexualities or those perceived as being in any way different from a perceived tough 'norm' of heterosexuality. Homophobia often makes up part of the 'macho' defensive armour for young men's developing masculinities. Fears about their own sexuality can be a reason for homophobia amongst boys (see Chapter 8 for discussion on young men and homophobia).

Bullying includes:

• deliberate hostility and aggression towards the victim
• a victim who is weaker and less powerful than the bully or bullies
• an outcome that is always painful and distressing for the victim.

Bullying can be physical, verbal, emotional, racist or sexual.

All incidents should be tackled with sensitivity and an understanding that the dynamics of the circumstances may be complicated. Any bullying incident that occurs and is reported should be acknowledged, dealt with promptly and recorded. As a visitor to the school, incidents should be reported to the teaching staff for appropriate follow-up according to their bullying policy.

Tips for tackling bullying during an outreach session

• The unacceptability of bullying should be highlighted at the beginning of the session and ideally included in the group agreement.

- Take immediate action when bullying is observed. As an adult and role model, you must let young people know that you care and will not allow anyone to be mistreated. By taking immediate action and dealing directly with the bully, adults support both the victim and the witnesses.
- Talk to bullies in private. Challenging a bully in front of their peers may actually enhance their status and lead to further aggression.
- Avoid attempts to mediate a bullying situation. The difference in power between victims and bullies may cause victims to feel further victimised by the process or believe that they are somehow at fault.

Evaluation

Evaluation is an important part of the outreach process. It provides the opportunity to assess whether skills have been learned and ensures that follow-up work for the group can be planned and amendments made to the programme. This process should involve both facilitators and young people. It helps to ensure the content of the session is relevant and responsive to the needs of the students and enables facilitators' training needs to be identified.

Evaluation should cover the most useful and least useful aspects of the session, the effectiveness of the facilitators and any changes that might improve the session. Participatory methods of evaluation can enable less verbal individuals to demonstrate what they have learned and understood. This feedback can be gathered via graffiti sheets, post-it notes or a process similar to the game of consequences, where students write their comments on a sheet then fold it over for the next person to write theirs.

As facilitator ask yourself:[6]

- Skills – what have they learned to do?
- Information – what do they now know?
- Attitudes and values – what do they think, feel, believe?
- Did girls and boys engage equally with the activity?
- What do they need to learn next?

Ask the young people to answer the questions:

- What new information have I learned?
- What new skills did I practise?
- How will I be able to use what I have learned?
- What else do I need to learn?

References

1 Swann C, Bowe K, McCormick G *et al.* (2003) *Teenage Pregnancy and Parenthood: a review of reviews.* Health Development Agency, London.
2 Family Planning Association Northern Ireland (2003) *Sex Education in Schools.* fpa, Belfast.
3 National Curriculum Council (1990) *National Curriculum Guidance 5: health education.* National Curriculum Council, London.

4   Department for Education and Employment (1996) *The Education Act 1996.* HMSO, London.

5   Stewart D and Ray C (2001) *Ensuring Entitlement: sex and relationships education for disabled children.* Sex Education Forum and the Council for Disabled Children, National Children's Bureau, London.

6   Sex Education Forum (1997) *Effective Learning: approaches to teaching sex education.* Factsheet 12. National Children's Bureau, London.

7   Sex Education Forum (1999) *Supporting Parents in Sex and Relationships Education.* Factsheet 18. National Children's Bureau, London.

8   www.sexualhealthsheffield.co.uk

9   Sex Education Forum (1997) *Supporting Boys and Young Men in Sex and Relationships Education.* Factsheet 11. National Children's Bureau, London.

10   City and Hackney SRE Team (2003) Contraception workshop. City and Hackney Primary Care Trust, London. Unpublished.

Resources

- *Department for Education and Employment circular 0016/2000*
  Outlines schools' duties regarding SRE provision.
  Available from Department for Education and Skills. Tel: 0845 6022260.
- Department of Health (2003) *Effective Sexual Health Promotion: a tool-kit for primary care trusts and others working in the field of promoting good sexual health and HIV prevention.* HMSO, London. www.doh.gov.uk/sexualhealthandhiv/toolkit.htm
- Lenderyou G (1993) *Primary School Sex Education Workbook: teaching sex education within the National Curriculum.* Family Planning Association, London.
- The Clarity Collective (1989) *Taught Not Caught.* London Development Agency, London.
- Lloyd K and Lyth N (2003) Evaluation of the use of drama in sex and relationship education. *Nursing Times.* **99** (47): 32–4.
- www.ncb.org.uk/sexed.htm
- Sex Education Forum website for a regularly updated list of resources.
- Sex Education Forum (1996) *Guidelines on the Effective Use of Outside Visitors in School Sex Education.* Factsheet 8. National Children's Bureau, London.
- Sex Education Forum (1999) *Supporting Parents in Sex and Relationships Education.* Factsheet 18. National Children's Bureau, London.
- Jewitt C (1994) *Exploring Healthy Sexuality: a guide to sex education in a youth setting.* Family Planning Association, London.
- *Nothing But The Facts: where to get help when you need it*
  A colourful, pocket-sized leaflet aimed at young people aged 14 and above. It provides practical advice on where to go to get help in confidence, and compares what's on offer at Brook Centres, young people's advisory clinics, doctors' surgeries and GUM clinics and what to expect when you walk through the door.
- www.brook.org.uk

Appendix 1: Connexions

Connexions is the Government's support service for all young people aged 13–19 in England. The service aims to provide integrated advice, guidance and access to personal development opportunities for this group and to help them make a smooth transition to adulthood and working life.

Connexions joins together the work of Government departments with private and voluntary sector groups and youth and careers services. It brings together all the services and support young people need during their teenage years. It offers practical help with choosing the right courses and careers, including access to broader personal development through activities such as sport, performing arts and volunteering activities. It also provides help and advice on issues such as drug abuse, sexual health and homelessness.

Connexions offers integrated support to young people. All young people will have access to a personal adviser. For some this may be just for careers advice, for others it may involve more in-depth support to help identify barriers to learning and find solutions and access to more specialist support. The personal advisers will work in a range of settings, including schools, colleges, one-stop shops and community centres, and on an outreach basis.

A national Connexions website contains information for personal advisers and other professionals: www.connexions.gov.uk. There is also a national Connexions website for young people: www.connexions-direct.com/. Connexions Direct can help with information and advice on issues relating to health, housing, relationships with family and friends, career and learning options, money, as well as activities to get involved in. There are also websites for local Connexions partnerships.

Appendix 2: *Framework for the Assessment of Children in Need and Their Families*

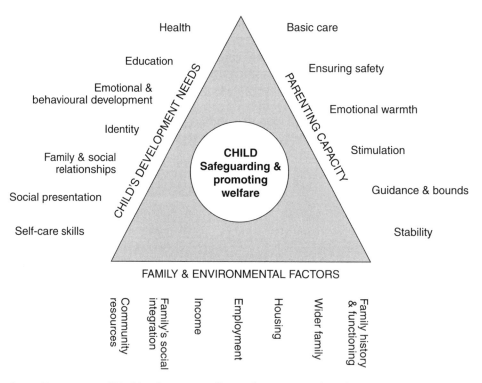

Source: Department of Health, The Home Office and Department.for Education and Employment (1999) *Working Together to Safeguard Children*. Department of Health/The Home Office/DfEE, London, page 112. *See also*: www.dh.gov.uk/assetRoot/04/07/58/24/04075824.pdf.

Appendix 3: Abortion

Abortion in England and Wales is legal as long as it follows the law set out in the Abortion Act 1967. This states that an abortion may be legally carried out if:

- two doctors agree that continuing the pregnancy would risk the life of the mother or risk injury to her physical or mental health
- two doctors agree that there is a substantial risk that the child might be born with a serious physical or mental handicap.

Abortion is not legal in Northern Ireland, apart from exceptional circumstances.

An abortion must by law (except in a few extreme cases) be carried out before week 24 of pregnancy.

If the young person is under 16, it is not necessary for parental consent as long as the young person is deemed competent to have medical treatment according to the Fraser Guidelines.

The father, whether he is married to the mother or not, has no right to prevent her from having a legal abortion.

A doctor does not have to refer a woman requesting an abortion if it is against their conscience. If that happens, they should arrange for the young woman to see another doctor.

Safety

Legal abortion is very safe for the woman. There is very little risk, particularly in early pregnancy. However, no clinical procedure is entirely free from risk. The doctor will explain these risks during the pre-abortion assessment. Early abortion is safe and does not affect a woman's chance of having a baby in the future.

There are two types of abortion: surgical and medical.

Surgical abortion

An early abortion is carried out by vacuum aspiration: the contents of the uterus are sucked out by an electric pump. This takes about 10–15 minutes and is usually done under a general anaesthetic. The client can usually go home on the same day.

Medical abortion

If a young woman is less than nine weeks' pregnant she can take tablets to stop the pregnancy. Two days later, in a hospital or clinic, the woman has a vaginal pessary that softens the cervix and lets the contents of the uterus out.

After the abortion most women experience an overwhelming sense of relief, although sometimes this is accompanied by feelings of sadness or guilt. The crisis of an unplanned pregnancy can evoke strong feelings and some women may benefit from counselling.

Appendix 4: Standard occupational class definitions

A	Upper middle class	Higher managerial, administrative or professional
B	Middle class	Intermediate managerial, administrative or professional
CI	Lower middle class	Supervisor or clerical
CII	Skilled working class	Skilled manual workers
D	Working class	Semi and unskilled manual workers
E	Those at lowest level of subsistence	State pensioners, etc. with no other earnings

Appendix 5: Sure Start

Sure Start is a government programme which aims to achieve better outcomes for children, parents and communities by:

- increasing the availability of childcare for all children
- improving emotional development for young children
- supporting parents as parents and in their aspirations towards employment.

This will be achieved by:

- helping services develop in disadvantaged areas alongside financial help for parents to afford childcare
- rolling out the principles driving the Sure Start approach to all services for children and parents.

www.surestart.gov.uk/aboutsurestart/

Appendix 6: Cervical screening

What is cervical screening?

Cervical screening is a method of preventing cancer by detecting and treating early abnormalities which, if left untreated, could lead to cancer in a woman's cervix (the neck of the womb).

Early detection and treatment can prevent 80–90% of cancers developing, but like other screening tests it is not perfect. It may not always detect early cell changes that could lead to cancer.

How is it done?

A cervical smear test can usually be done very quickly and easily, either by a trained nurse or doctor. It involves an internal examination.

A speculum is inserted to open out the walls of the vagina a little so that the nurse or doctor can see the cervix. Then, using a flat wooden or plastic spatula, some loose cells are scraped off the cervix and transferred to a microscope slide or a bottle. This is then sent to the laboratory where the cells are examined.

Women are usually informed of the results by post directly from the laboratory or regional smear testing service. If the results are abnormal the woman may be called back for a repeat smear a few weeks later. Often mild cell changes get better on their own. Some women are referred directly back to see a specialist because cell changes are more serious.

Who is entitled to the screening?

Cervical screening is offered to women aged between 25 and 65. The first invitation is automatically issued at 25; three-yearly smears are offered between the ages of 25 and 49, and five-yearly between 50 and 64.

Cervical cancer is rare in women under 20. Teenagers' bodies, particularly the cervix, are still developing, which means young women may get an abnormal smear result when there is nothing wrong. This could lead to unnecessary investigations and treatment, causing unnecessary worry.

Under the age of 25 years invasive cancer is extremely rare, but changes in the cervix are common. Although lesions treated in very young women may prevent cancers from developing many years later, the evidence suggests that the best time to begin screening is age 25. Lesions that are destined to progress will still be screen-detectable and those that would regress will no longer be a source of anxiety.

Women aged 65 and over who have had three consecutive negative smears are taken out of the recall system. The natural history and progression of cervical cancer means it is highly unlikely that such women will go on to develop the disease. Women aged 65 and over who have never had a smear are entitled to a test.

If a woman has never been sexually active with a man, the research evidence shows that her chance of developing cervical cancer is very low.

(www.cancerscreening.nhs.uk/cervical/publications/in-04.html)

Results

The cytologist examining the slide will look for pre-cancerous changes in the cells known as dyskaryosis or dysplasia. There are four types: borderline, mild, moderate and severe.

About 50% of women with mild dysplasia will have their changes revert to normal after six months, so these women will be asked to have a repeat smear six months later. If mild changes persist on the second smear, they will undergo further assessment by colposcopy.

Women with smears showing moderate or severe pre-cancerous changes will be referred for colposcopy as they have a significant risk of proceeding to cervical cancer if left untreated.

Colposcopy

After a woman has had an abnormal cervical smear, it is necessary to examine her cervix with a microscope or colposcope. The woman sits on a special couch which supports her legs and a speculum is passed to visualise the cervix (just like having a smear).

Tissue analysis by the pathologist divides pre-cancerous changes into low-grade or high-grade squamous intraepithelial lesions (SIL). If the abnormality occupies the first third of the cervical skin it is called CIN I (cervical intraepithelial neoplasia), and two thirds, CIN II. If the pre-cancerous cells occupy the full thickness it is called CIN III – the old name for this was 'carcinoma *in situ*'.

For women who have CIN II, CIN III or persistent CIN I pre-cancerous changes, the most common treatment is called Large Loop Excision of the Transformation Zone (LLETZ), also called Loop Electro-Excision Procedure (LEEP).

A loop of wire through which an electric current flows is used to shave off the abnormal cells. Like a tiny cheese wire, the loop cuts out the abnormal piece of skin from the cervix and seals up the area as it passes through. Any residual abnormal tissue can be destroyed by another pass of the loop or more cautery. The client can have local or general anaesthesia.

After treatment there is usually a colposcopy examination and cervical smear four to six months later which begins a programme of regular surveillance.

(www.colposcopy.org.uk/)

Appendix 7:
Clinical supervision

Clinical supervision is defined as:

> A formal process of professional support and learning which enables individual practitioners to develop knowledge and competence, assume responsibility for their own practice, and enhance consumer protection and safety of care in complex clinical situations. It is central to the process of learning and to the scope of the expansion of practice and should be seen as a means of encouraging self-assessment and analytical and reflective skills.

(www.clinical-supervision.com)

Appendix 8: Sample confidentiality policy

Confidentiality Policy

- Confidentiality is central to the work of everyone working with young people.
- All information about clients is confidential.
- The duty of confidentiality owed to a person under 16 is as great as the duty owed to any other person.
- All clients can expect that their personal information will not be disclosed without their permission except in the most exceptional circumstances, when someone is at risk of serious harm.

Staff responsibilities
- All professionals must follow their professional codes of practice and the law. This means that they must make every effort to protect confidentiality.
- All professionals are individually accountable for their own actions. They should work together as a team to ensure that standards of confidentiality are upheld and that improper disclosures are avoided.
- Standards of confidentiality apply to all professionals, administrative and ancillary staff, and also to students or others observing practice. They must not reveal to anybody outside the service personal information they learn in the course of their work or through their presence in the clinic without the patient's consent. Nor will they discuss with colleagues any aspect of a client's attendance at the clinic in a way that might allow identification of the client, unless doing so is necessary for the client's care.

If disclosure is necessary
- If a client or another person is at grave risk of serious harm, the professional will counsel the client about the benefits of disclosure. If the client refuses to allow disclosure, the professional can take advice from colleagues within the service, or from a professional, regulatory or defence body, in order to decide whether a disclosure without consent is justified to protect the patient or another person. If a decision is taken to disclose, the client should always be informed before the disclosure is made, unless to do so could be dangerous. If possible, any such decisions should be shared with another member of the team.
- Any decision to disclose information to protect health, safety or well-being will be based on the degree of current or potential harm, not on the age of the patient.

Appendix 9: Sample child protection policy

Child Protection Policy

This policy applies to all staff working in the clinic. There are five main elements to this policy:

1 ensuring safe recruitment in checking the suitability of staff and volunteers to work with children
2 raising awareness of child protection issues and equipping children with the skills needed to keep them safe
3 developing and then implementing procedures for identifying and reporting cases, or suspected cases, of abuse
4 supporting young people who have been abused
5 establishing a safe environment for young people.

It is recognised that because of the nature of the work (sexual health advice and services) clinic staff are well placed to observe the outward signs of abuse. The team will therefore strive to establish and maintain an environment where young people feel secure, are encouraged to talk, and are listened to.

All staff will follow the procedures set out by the Area Child Protection Committee and take account of guidance issued by the Department of Health to:

- ensure there is a designated member of staff for child protection who has received appropriate training and support for this role
- ensure every member of staff knows the name of the designated staff member responsible for child protection and their role
- ensure all staff understand their responsibilities in being alert to the signs of abuse and for referring any concerns to the designated staff member responsible for child protection
- develop effective links with relevant agencies and cooperate as required with their enquiries regarding child protection matters, including attendance at case conferences
- keep written records of concerns about children, even where there is no need to refer the matter immediately
- ensure all records are kept securely in locked locations.

Appendix 10:
Integrated care pathways

An integrated care pathway is defined as follows:

> An integrated care pathway brings together all the anticipated elements of care and treatment of all members of the multidisciplinary team, for a patient or client of a particular case type or grouping within an agreed time frame, for the achievement of agreed outcomes. Any deviation from the plan is documented as a 'variance'; the analysis of which provides information for the review of current practice.

(Johnson S (1997) *Pathways of Care*. Blackwell Science, Oxford)

Appendix 11: The National Healthy School Standard

What is the National Healthy School Standard?

Jointly funded by the Department for Education and Skills and the Department of Health, the National Healthy School Standard is part of the Government's drive to reduce health inequalities, promote social inclusion and raise educational standards. The overall aim is to help schools become healthier.

A healthy school is one that is successful in helping pupils do their best and build on their achievements. It is committed to ongoing improvement and development. It promotes physical and emotional health by providing accessible and relevant information and equipping pupils with the skills and attitudes to make informed decisions about their health. A healthy school understands the importance of investing in health to assist in the process of raising levels of pupil achievement and improving standards. It also recognises the need to provide both physical and social environments that are conducive to learning.

What does the National Healthy School Standard say about sex and relationships education?

- The school should have a policy which is owned and implemented by all members of the school, including pupils and parents, and which is delivered in partnership with local health and support services.
- The school should have a planned sex and relationships education programme (including information, social skills development and values clarification) which identifies learning outcomes appropriate to pupils' age, ability, gender and level of maturity and which is based on pupils' needs assessment and a knowledge of vulnerable pupils.
- Staff should have a sound basic knowledge of sex and relationships issues and be confident in their skills to teach sex education and discuss sex and relationships.
- Staff should have an understanding of the role of schools in contributing to the reduction of unwanted teenage conceptions and the promotion of sexual health.

(Department for Education and Employment (1999)
National Healthy School Standard Guidance. HMSO, London)

Appendix 12: Sex and relationships education (National Curriculum guidance, 1999)

The Sex and Relationships Education Guidance states that sex and relationships education (SRE) should be firmly rooted within the framework for personal, social and health education (PSHE) and citizenship.

There is specific National Curriculum guidance for the sex and relationships education programme, which is summarised below.

Key stage 3 (age 11–14, school years 7–9)
PSHE

- To reflect on and assess their strengths in relation to personality, work and leisure. To respect the differences between people as they develop their own sense of identity.
- To recognise the stages of emotions associated with loss and change caused by death, divorce, separation and new family members, and how to deal positively with the strength of their feelings in different situations.
- To recognise the physical and emotional changes that take place at puberty and how to manage these in a positive way.
- In the context of the importance of relationships, to know about human reproduction, contraception, sexually transmitted infections, HIV and high-risk behaviours, including early sexual activity.
- To know about the effects of all types of stereotyping, prejudice, bullying, racism and discrimination and how to challenge them assertively.
- To explore how to empathise with people different from themselves.
- To explore the nature of friendship and how to make and keep friends.
- To recognise some of the cultural norms in society, including the range of lifestyles and relationships.
- To explore the changing nature of, and pressure on, relationships with friends and family, and when and how to seek help.
- To discuss the role and importance of marriage in family relationships.
- To know about the roles and feelings of parents and carers and the values of family life.

- To recognise that goodwill is essential to positive and constructive relationships.
- To negotiate within relationships, recognising that actions have consequences and when and how to make compromises.
- To resist pressure to do wrong, and to recognise when others need help and how to support them.
- To communicate confidently with their peers and adults.

Science

- To learn about the physical and emotional changes that take place during adolescence.
- To know about the human reproductive system, including the menstrual cycle and fertilisation.
- To know how the fetus develops in the uterus, including the role of the placenta.

Key stage 4 (age 15–16, school years 10–11)
PSHE

- To have a sense of their own identity and present themselves confidently in a range of situations.
- To recognise influences, pressures and sources of help and respond to them appropriately.
- To think about the alternatives and long- and short-term consequences when making decisions about personal health.
- To use assertiveness skills to resist unhelpful pressure.
- To seek professional advice confidently and find information about health.
- To be aware of exploitation in relationships.
- To challenge offending behaviour, prejudice, bullying, racism and discrimination assertively and take the initiative in giving and receiving support.
- To be able to talk about relationships and feelings.
- To deal with changing relationships in a positive way, showing goodwill to others and using strategies to resolve disagreements peacefully.
- To discuss the nature and importance of marriage for family life and bringing up children.
- To know about the statutory and voluntary organisations that support relationships in crisis.

Index